The Exercise Myth

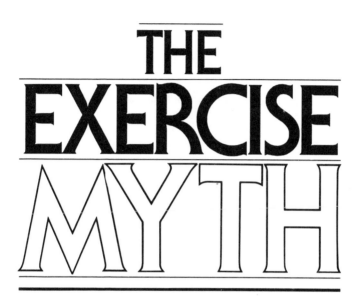

THE EXERCISE MYTH

Henry A. Solomon, M.D.

HARCOURT BRACE JOVANOVICH, PUBLISHERS

SAN DIEGO   NEW YORK   LONDON

Library of Congress Cataloging in Publication Data
Solomon, Henry A.
The exercise myth.
Bibliography: p.
Includes index.
1. Exercise. 2. Exercise—Physiological aspects.
I. Title.
RA781.S6225   1983   613.7'1   83-22672
ISBN 0-15-129458-5

Designed by Jacqueline Schuman
Printed in the United States of America
First edition
A B C D E

HBJ

To my family, whose encouragement and
forbearance made this book possible.

To my friends and patients, whose interest
and enthusiasm spurred me and for whom my
respect, affection and concern are boundless.

Contents

The Exercise Myth

1
The Exercise Marketplace

I see them early in the morning on my way to work. I see them from my office windows during the day. And in the evening, they are still hustling back and forth: women in stylish gear hurrying to exercise class; middle-aged men huffing to and from Central Park; people of every age and description panting and sweating their way to today's version of the healthy lifestyle.

I am a cardiologist, as eager to save others' lives as they are to hold on to their own. And yet for all my concern and their effort, exercisers are as likely as any to wind up among my patients. Those exercisers I get to see, and perhaps to help, are only a few of the tens of millions in the United States who now run or jog regularly, and the merest fraction of those many millions more in this country and around the world who have taken up the banner of vigorous exercise in general. They are the representatives of all those who have bought the mistaken idea that strenuous effort promotes health and longevity. They

1

seek an unattainable goal. They are the victims of the exercise myth.

No one knows exactly how many individuals exercise hard and often in the belief that they are doing themselves good. Although there are probably millions of believers who work out in gyms, on handball courts, at tennis clubs, in dance classes and other meeting grounds, runners are today the most visible of those who incorporate vigorous and often punishing exercise into their everyday lives. You can get an impression, at least, of how many joggers doggedly pound the pavement of city streets or trot the shoulders of suburban roads by just looking around you during the popular early-morning and after-work hours. Their number has been guessed to be 30 million.

More reliable numbers exist for "real" runners—those who run marathons or enter lesser races. There are now about 300 organized marathons run yearly around the world. Fred Lebow, president of the New York Road Runners Club, refers to "marathon fever" in describing the spread of such organized racing. The Boston Marathon has about 8,000 registered entrants; another 8,000 unregistered runners—the registered racers call them "bandits"—usually join the race. The last L'Eggs Mini-Marathon, a 6.4-mile race in New York City, registered about 6,500 women from 34 states and 8 countries. The increasingly popular Montreal Marathon now has about 10,000 entrants, and the New York Marathon, perhaps the most famous race of all, now attracts about 17,000 registrants. One would have to guess that there are hundreds—maybe thousands—of "mere" joggers or novice runners to every registered racer. And there must be at least as many people who strive for their weekly dose of exercise in other ways.

In former days, the healthiest form of exercise was thought to be a daily "constitutional"—a modestly brisk walk that could be accomplished without special gear and certainly without panting. We've come a long way, but why? Runners run and exercisers exercise because so many people have told them it's good for them physically, emotionally, socially and even spiritually. The distinctions between various benefits are rather blurred to judge by the books and magazines that promote exercise. *Self*, a smashing success on the newsstands these days, is described by its editor as a magazine of "physical and emotional well-being." The titles of other new entries into the field—*New Body, American Health, Shape, Fit, Spring*—promise a blend of radiant skin, lithe figure, athletic prowess and excellent health. Traditional magazines, whether devoted to motherhood or fashion, have dramatically altered their format and thrust to reflect the new emphasis on exercise.

Social pressure to participate in the movement is quite real. You're as likely to hear mention of "aerobics" and "cardiovascular fitness" in cocktail-party conversation as you are to hear about the latest theatrical hit, new restaurant or fashion news. And you're expected to respond with the right knowledge, jargon and enthusiasm.

Knowledge and jargon aren't hard to come by. Bookstore shelves are filled with exercise books, treatises on how to run and when to run, on strengthening your body, on changing it and making it better. The enthusiasm is catching. *Jane Fonda's Workout Book* was number one on the *New York Times* bestseller list for 51 weeks—in some spot on the list for 92 weeks—and James Fixx's best-selling book[1] on running sold nearly 1 million copies in hardcover alone. Its author, who said he could "show you how to become healthier and happier than you ever imagined you could be,"* became highly visible in television commercials.

Strong business and career pressures are often exerted to

* The notes are on pages 136–143.

3

make people conform to the dogma of the exercise believers. Subtle—and not-so-subtle—influences may compel otherwise unwilling individuals to participate in physical-activity programs. In 1980, over 3,000 businesses were providing health/fitness programs for employees. Some corporations have made large financial investments in building their own exercise facilities for the use of all their personnel. Other companies pay considerable sums of money to outside exercise facilities for their executives, and individual participation in the programs may be periodically reviewed. *Runners Handbook* reported that in one major corporation, employees who don't exercise are gently admonished by their colleagues. No wonder; $5 billion is spent yearly on employee-fitness programs,[2] and no business likes to see its investments wasted.

The Corporate Challenge Series has become, except for the New York Marathon, the largest race organized by the New York Road Runners Club. It receives a lot of media attention, and competition, while friendly, is intense. The latest Corporate Challenge race attracted 8,000 runners. As described by Deborah Greene, race director of the 1980 Manufacturers Hanover Corporate Challenge, in *New York Running News*, "after a hard day at the office, tired corporate workers, from office boys to presidents, wended their way toward Central Park . . . for a competitive race. They came dressed to run, parading the streets in shorts, running shoes, and singlets emblazoned with the names of their companies. They . . . huddled under the signs or banners of their corporate teams."[3]

Whether facilities and programs for exercise and competition are fostered by true but misplaced benevolent concern on the part of corporate management or by the unproven expectation and hope of greater employee productivity, the fact is that the manager or executive who doesn't see these corporate commitments as an unspoken corporate philosophy or command may be risking career advancement. Within one's business world, as within one's neighborhood, being "into" exercise undeniably conveys a certain status.

Television has had an important influence on the fitness phenomenon. The glorification of winners and the intense publicity surrounding what are largely media events—the runner has been called the "darling of the media"—allow even the amateur to feel special. Whereas regular network television blazed the trail by increasing coverage of the professional and trained athlete, cable television focuses heavily on the untrained amateur, that person at home who could be you. The Cable Health Network, for example, is a relatively new twenty-four-hour cable television channel dealing only with health and fitness. A wide range of programs is broadcast, with the heaviest emphasis on exercise.

The consensus that exercise is beneficial—reflected in the social, career and media pressures to exercise, and the coupling of fitness to health, beauty, sexual, social and business success—is both the product of, and the impetus for, a variety of extravagant and unfounded claims about what exercise can do for you. Many promise medical help. A highly successful exercise center in New York offers a "systematic program designed to strengthen your heart . . . and help reduce coronary risk factors. . . ." A professional dancer offers a course in aerobics that will "strengthen your cardiovascular system . . ." and have you "thoroughly enjoy your return to good health and a good figure." A nationwide network of rehabilitation centers for cardiac patients promotes "safe, supervised, telemetry-monitored exercise therapy . . ." through which "you'll find a new way of life . . . an atmosphere of hope, not heartbreak." Even a manufacturer of corn oil offers an "information-packed booklet" in which "different types of exercises are evaluated for fitness and cardiovascular health." And a dentist suggests that you "jog over" to his office for special "dentistry for the runner."

Promises of medical help often tend to shade into promises of spiritual renewal. One exercise center coins a new term, "biofitness," and offers "a tailormade program, based on individual needs, to integrate the mind and body in a get-well-get-better goal."

Perhaps the exaggeration of benefits and blurring of claims are best summed up in the advertisement of a large sporting-goods store, which promises that its indoor jogging treadmill fosters "Cardiovascular Health, Aerobic Fitness, Facilitates Sleep, Better Balance, Muscle Strength, Feeling of Euphoria, Better Health, Increased Stamina, Weight Control."

No wonder people are willing to pay for such a panacea. And pay they do. On the basis of amazing claims, the public is spending enormous sums of money for exercise clothing, equipment and programs, and exercise has become very big business. On Wall Street, it would be called a "growth industry." Sales of jogging shoes, for example, have more than doubled in the last five years, although some may buy them more for comfort or style than for running. One out of every three pairs of shoes sold in the United States is sneakers. The Nike Company alone sold about 13 million running shoes in 1983; and their total sales, now including other apparel as well as shoes, are in the hundreds of millions of dollars. The sheer number of different running shoes is astounding. A few years ago, a leading runners' magazine listed about a dozen brands. The latest available report lists over one hundred. The number of models must be staggering.

The National Sporting Goods Association estimated 1982 sales to individuals (not counting any institutional sales) of athletic equipment, including barbells, treadmills, trampolines, exercise bicycles, rowing machines and jump ropes, to be $499.4 million. Individuals bought 42.2 million pairs of exercise shorts for $374 million. They spent $212 million on sweat shirts, and $385 million on warm-up suits. Thomas B. Doyle, director of information and research for the association, calls these figures conservative, and estimates they are 25 percent lower than actual sales figures.

In keeping with the coupling of exercise to beauty, status and success, the business of clothing exercisers is high fashion by now. The term "locker-room chic" has been coined and is actually the name of the fashion section of a new magazine. Warm-up suits, running shorts, socks, shirts, hats, visors, sunglasses, headbands, are all promoted via an ingeniously successful amalgam of fashion and fitness.

Runners and other exercisers are just as trendy and slavish to fashion as anyone else. Of course, much of the fashion emphasis has been directed to women, and a number of new products have been created to capitalize on the demand. Since the number of women athletes has increased greatly, manufacturers have introduced more than a dozen "sports bras" in the past few years. "Joggers' bounce" and "joggers' nipples" are now terms of common parlance. "Whatever your sport," one brand claims, "there's a bra. . . ." They offer the racquet bra and the active-woman exercise bra, as well as the running bra.

Most believers in exercise deny that their devotion to physical activity is greatly influenced by advertising promotion, social or career considerations. They claim to be immune to such blandishments despite the money spent on "selling" exercise through the allure of its association with beauty and success. My own observations suggest otherwise. And, anyway, getting together on the courts or on the running track probably does have some social benefits, just as exercise among executives and business people probably does offer career benefits. Ultimately, though, exercisers offer a more hard-nosed reason for their devotion. They believe that vigorous, even punishing exercise

7

leads to better health and longer life. They believe, specifically, that exercise promotes cardiovascular health and protects against heart attack, the leading cause of death in this country and in other industrialized societies.

The idea of immunity from cardiovascular disease by virtue of vigorous exercise has been the foundation upon which interest and participation in exercise have grown. Achieving a longer life and a healthier one through exercise is the single constant thread woven through the history of the recent exercise revolution.

This is my concern—the claims of longevity, improved cardiovascular health and immunity to heart disease. As a physician, I may hold a personal opinion about the social fringe benefits of exercise, but not a professional one. As a physician, however, I ought to have a professional opinion about health in general. And as a cardiologist, I must, and do, have a strong opinion about the specific relationship of exercise to cardiovascular health and longevity.

Physicians have had a major role in the growth and maturing of the exercise revolution. Whether the medical profession really started the exercise craze or simply joined the growing movement is arguable. Doctors have certainly put their own muscle behind the exercise bandwagon and enthusiastically leaped aboard as it got rolling. The medical profession provides a legitimacy for exercise where otherwise there would be none. Science is thought somehow to be above faddism, and physicians' interests are thought to be purely scientific. When doctors sanction the exercise revolution, the accompanying commitments of money and time, as well as any risks to health and safety, then become acceptable.

The first major medical reference to the potential health-promoting qualities of exercise was a study of London transit workers conducted by Jeremy Noah Morris, of the Medical

Research Council, London Hospital. In an article entitled "Coronary Heart Disease and Physical Activity of Work," published in 1953 in the English medical journal *Lancet*, Morris and his colleagues compared the amount and severity of coronary heart disease in London bus drivers and in bus conductors. They observed that the more sedentary drivers had more coronary disease than did the more active conductors. They concluded that physical activity offers protection from coronary heart disease.[4]

There was no great public reaction to the appearance of this technical paper in a scientific journal, but it had considerable impact on the medical profession, which saw in it a new glimmer of hope for the prevention of heart disease. To this day, Morris's study is considered a landmark, its conclusions well known to most physicians.

After the publication of Morris's original paper, a steady stream of articles concerning the possible health benefits of physical activity began to appear in medical journals, keeping exercise as a topic of medical concern at a high level. Meanwhile, a diagnostic test was coming into common use, and it lulled doctors into believing they could thereby diagnose the condition of a patient's heart, and could even tell whether exercise was safe for that person. This was the Master Two-Step Test, named for its developer, Dr. Arthur M. Master, of New York City, who introduced the test in about 1925 and later reported his results in leading medical journals.

The idea underlying this first stress test was that abnormalities of the heart that were not apparent at rest could become evident under conditions of physical stress. In other words, physical stress—exercise—could provoke abnormal cardiac responses. Since the heart works harder during activity, physical effort could be used to bring out heart trouble. Conversely, if physical stress did not provoke abnormalities, then the patient's heart could be considered normal. The logical corollary was that a normal performance on the stress test meant that physical exercise was safe.

As time went on, refinements in exercise stress testing were made. In addition to the simple steps used in the Master Two-Step Test, treadmills and exercise bicycles were developed. A steady promotional effort began to be directed at physicians. Many new companies manufacturing exercise testing and monitoring devices sprang up. Soon, the age of computer-assisted and computer-directed stress testing arrived. The newer devices are highly sophisticated and complex compared with the original Two-Step device, and convey a much greater sense of diagnostic precision and accuracy. Manufacturing and marketing efforts today are stronger than ever.

If the science and technology of modern-day stress testing are somewhat confusing, even to many physicians, the financial incentives are clearer. Since stress testing is a complicated and potentially risky procedure, and does take time, fees are high. An exercise stress test in New York City, for example, may easily cost between $150 and $250. To many physicians, fees from stress testing in its various forms represent a significant percentage of their total income. The marketing efforts of companies selling exercise testing equipment to physicians almost always prominently feature the economic rewards to be gained. Every sales effort ever made to me by a company selling exercise equipment has emphasized how quickly I can earn back the cost. The company even provides an analysis showing just how few tests per month are needed to break even, and then how many to earn multiples of the purchase price. And since third-party payers—Blue Shield and other health insurance providers—cover much of the cost of the tests, financial considerations rarely dissuade patients from having the tests done.

More entrepreneurial individuals, recognizing that increased volume means increased revenues, have established exercise testing centers. People come on their own or are referred by physicians or exercise clinics for stress testing. These exercise testing centers are often owned outright by physicians. Alternatively, physicians may have equity positions, usually in exchange for serving as "consultants" or "advisers."

Stress testing is actually only a small part of the financial reward from these exercise centers. "Supervised" exercise programs represent a much greater financial return. More and more, cardiac patients are being advised to participate in regular exercise programs. Since some 350,000 people survive heart attacks each year and there are altogether several million cardiac patients in the United States, the potential "pool" of subjects is very large. Most exercise testing centers also run supervised exercise programs; the revenue potential is obvious.

More than 20 "cardiac rehabilitation clinics" opened on Long Island, New York, alone in the last few years. As the field of exercise testing and supervised exercise programs gets crowded and competition is felt, one way to help insure a successful operation has been to divide ownership among several physicians, who then have an incentive to recommend the program to their patients. One such center admits, according to the *New York Times*, that 85 percent of the program's patients come from shareholder physicians.

Of course, not every physician who recommends exercise does it out of venality or solely for profit. Doctors themselves participate in vigorous workouts and demanding games. At many medical meetings there are running groups who are accorded special status. One major pharmaceutical company sponsors mini-marathons for physicians and their spouses at varous medical conventions. These races feature trophies and awards, and, as a company spokesman puns, "are just for the health of it." Doctors, despite their medical training, are consumers just like everyone else, subject to the same exercise ballyhoo and hype as the rest of the population.

So, everything has come together. The enticement of profit, the seductions of fashion and status, and the legitimacy of medicine all support this amazing exercise phenomenon. So huge a bandwagon, fueled by the profit motive and weighted by a population worried about its health and believing it has found the answer, has a terrible momentum. The sober truth may not be enough to stop it, but the truth should be stated:

You may enjoy exercise; it may be helpful socially; it may make you look and feel better. But all the rest is myth.

Exercise will not make you healthy. It will not make you live longer. Fitness and health are not the same thing.

2
The Heart of the Matter

Most of us respond easily to the common greeting "How are you?" because we have an intuitive sense that how we feel is, in fact, how we are. If we feel well, we answer that we're fine, and if we don't feel well, we may reply that we are not well. This intuitive merging of how we feel and how we are, however, is quite often incorrect.

Even in a strictly medical setting, people may mistakenly equate how they feel with their actual state of health. When I ask a patient "How do you feel?," I am seeking specific information about symptoms. When patients reply, as they sometimes half-jokingly do, "You tell me; you're the doctor," I say, "You tell me how you feel; I'll tell you how you are." The point—and it is a crucial one—is that how we feel is not necessarily how we are. How you are is a statement of your health, and has to do with the presence or absence of disease or abnormal body conditions. How you feel is a complex summation of physical, mental and emotional factors that is often independent of your actual state of health.

With regard to cardiovascular health, the divergence between how we feel and how we are may be especially striking. And the implications of this discrepancy between feeling and actuality can be serious. How we feel is largely dependent on what we can physically do—what is called "fitness"—but how we are may have little or nothing to do with this. Fitness and health are distinct and independent of one another.

Fitness is defined by your ability to do physical activity or to perform physical work. It is a measure of your "functional capacity." It doesn't reflect the presence or absence of disease, and implies nothing about the actual health of your arteries or your heart. Cardiovascular health refers to the absence of disease of the heart and blood vessels, not to the ability of an individual to do a certain amount of physical work. Your overall cardiac health is determined by the condition of various heart structures, including the heart muscle, the valves, the special cardiac tissues that carry electrical impulses and the coronary arteries. The health of coronary arteries has been claimed to be related to exercise.

Coronary arteries are those that carry oxygenated blood to the heart muscle. Healthy arteries are smooth-walled and of sufficient diameter inside for blood to flow freely through them. In coronary artery disease, or coronary heart disease, the arteries that carry blood to the heart muscle are narrowed and obstructed by deposits, called plaques, of cholesterol and other fatty substances. The heart muscle cells, like all other cells in the body, require oxygen to do their work. The heart doesn't get its oxygen from the blood inside it but from the network of coronary arteries that travel over and through the heart muscle. The pathologic process whereby the artery walls fill up with fatty substances and thereby narrow the channel through which

14

blood flows is called "atherosclerosis." It is the major abnormality in what is commonly called "hardening of the arteries." Since all of the oxygen carried to the body tissues travels in the blood, anything that decreases blood flow decreases oxygen supply. When coronary arteries are blocked or narrowed by atherosclerosis, not enough blood and therefore not enough oxygen reach heart muscle cells.

Coronary heart disease can be "silent" and produce no symptoms, or it can manifest itself in several ways, of which the most common are: the chest pain and breathlessness of angina pectoris, the even scarier event of a heart attack and—and this may be the first "symptom"—sudden death. These are about equally common as the first way coronary artery disease makes its presence known. By the time one of these occurs, the pathologic process of atherosclerosis has probably been going on for some time.

Angina pectoris literally means "strangling in the breast." Those words accurately describe the constricting chest pain that grips a person when there is a temporarily inadequate blood supply to heart muscle cells. Not every patient has this typical symptom, however. The person may instead feel less crushing pain, a sensation of burning or pressure, as well as breathlessness, weakness, faintness or fatigue. During an angina attack, when blood and oxygen supply are less than the heart needs, heart muscle cells are temporarily injured. If the blood and the oxygen supply are increased, or the heart muscle's need for blood and oxygen decreases, then the cells recover from injury and the symptoms go away completely.

A heart attack, known medically as a "myocardial infarction," represents actual death of some heart muscle cells. When a coronary artery is so narrowed that the blood supply is virtually cut off to an area of the heart muscle, the severely oxygen-deprived heart muscle cells are permanently injured and die.

Angina pectoris and heart attacks are really part of the same problem, but in angina the blood and the oxygen supply are not so inadequate relative to the heart muscle's needs as they are in a heart attack. Most initial heart attacks are not fatal, but if they are extensive enough or cause severe irregularities of the heart rhythm, they can cause death. Subsequent heart attacks are often more dangerous because the new damage is superimposed on the old.

Sudden cardiac death, the third common manifestation of coronary heart disease, is usually due to an arrhythmia, or irregularity of the heartbeat. There are many kinds of innocuous arrhythmias, and many normal people have them. Only one type of arrhythmia is usually quickly fatal. It almost always occurs in people with some serious form of heart disease, most usually coronary artery disease.

These three expressions of coronary artery disease—angina pectoris, heart attack and sudden cardiac death—are by no means mutually exclusive. Angina pectoris, for example, often precedes a heart attack, although it may first occur following one. Sudden cardiac death may happen without warning, but it also often follows a heart attack. And all these expressions— or none of them—may occur in any patient with coronary heart disease. But these indications of the underlying condition of the heart and its arteries have no relation to fitness. People with coronary heart disease and no symptoms, those with angina pectoris and heart attacks and those who will experience sudden cardiac death may all be in fine shape as far as their ability to exert themselves is concerned. Furthermore, almost no matter what their level of fitness, they may all enhance their functional capacity by exercise, yet the condition of their heart remains the same.

The fact that health and fitness are distinct, that people with severe, even imminently fatal coronary heart disease can be very fit and that individuals with coronary disease can enhance their functional capacity by exercise without thereby improving their health may be difficult to accept. The fact becomes more acceptable, however, with an understanding of what fitness is, and what the heart has to do with it.

The amount of physical work you can do—your fitness—ultimately depends on the amount of oxygen that your body tissues receive and can use. Functional capacity, in fact, is defined by physiologists in terms of oxygen utilization or oxygen consumption. The more oxygen your body can use, the more activity you can do; and the more physical work you actually do, the more oxygen your body consumes. Your ultimate fitness or functional capacity, then, is measured by the greatest amount of oxygen your body can use when you are performing at peak effort.

Since all of the oxygen your body tissues receive is carried in your bloodstream, and since the blood is pumped around your body by your heart, it seems intuitively logical that your functional capacity must depend primarily upon your heart. An increase in your capacity for physical work seems to imply an increase in the performance of your heart. As a logical consequence of a presumed enhancement of your heart's performance, the notions of a "stronger heart," "healthier heart" and "better heart" seem eminently sensible; certainly those notions have become uncritically accepted.

Your heart and cardiovascular system, however, are not always logical. What seems sensible and appears reasonable is not necessarily so. The fact of the matter is that much of what constitutes an improvement in your ability to perform physical work is *not* directly related to your heart. Although cardiac changes do occur as functional capacity increases, they are *not* inherently "better" or "healthier."

Since the amount of oxygen your body can use determines

your capacity for physical work, your body's fitness is limited by the amount of oxygen available to it. This, in turn, depends upon the amount of oxygen in the air you breathe, and on the condition of your lungs and your blood. Oxygen is transferred from the air to your bloodstream inside your lungs; diseases of the lungs or abnormalities in the blood itself can inhibit this normal transfer of oxygen from the air into your body.

Assuming the air you breathe has normal amounts of oxygen and you have no unusual lung or blood condition that interferes with oxygen entering your bloodstream, the amount of oxygen your body has available to it then depends upon how much blood your heart pumps to your cells. Your heart can increase the amount of blood it pumps around your body by increasing the "heart rate"—the number of heartbeats per minute—or by increasing what is called the "stroke volume"—the amount of blood pumped with each heartbeat. Assuming the heart is pumping plenty of blood around your body, how much oxygen can be used ultimately depends on the body cells. Your body cells can increase the amount of oxygen they use by extracting more of the available oxygen from the blood that comes to them.

Whenever you exercise or perform physical work, your body normally responds in a number of different ways. The most important of these changes, leading to increased oxygen availability to the body's cells in response to exertion, are increases in your heart rate and stroke volume. These increases are mainly due to nerve signals that your brain sends to your heart as more oxygen is needed. The combined effect of the heart changes is to pump more blood and thereby make more oxygen available to the cells of your body. But, additionally, removal of oxygen from the bloodstream by your body's muscle cells increases, since cells that produce and release energy at high rates, like working muscle cells, extract a large portion of the oxygen from the blood. All three effects—the increases in heart rate, stroke

18

volume and oxygen extraction—combine to allow you to do more activity.

If you exercise regularly at a certain intensity and for a certain period of time, you can achieve what has been called the "training effect." The term refers to a series of physiologic changes that occur in the body as a result of doing regular "aerobic" exercise. (Aerobic really just means "oxygen-using," and therefore all human activity is aerobic; applied to exercise, however, aerobic refers specifically to activity in which the amount of oxygen used by the body increases directly and predictably with the amount of physical exertion.) These physiologic changes of the training effect include: slower resting heart rate when you're inactive; slower heart rate and lower blood pressure when you're exerting at your peak level; faster return to your normal resting heart rate after you've finished exercising.

Somehow the notion mistakenly arose that these physiologic changes of the training effect are automatically "healthier" or "better." But there's no evidence that a slower resting heart rate is healthier than a heart rate somewhat faster, or that a quicker return to resting heart rate after exercise is inherently beneficial. Nobody has shown any biological advantage to a slower heartbeat. I have patients in their eighties and nineties who have somewhat rapid heartbeats and have had them since their childhoods. If you were born with a finite number of heartbeats for your lifetime, then a slower heart rate would be desirable, since you would live longer before using up your allotment. But there is no such allotted number of heartbeats for anybody.

Slower heart rate and lower blood pressure at physical exertion levels less than your maximum could possibly be advantageous. This would be so if you had a heart condition like angina pectoris, and physical activity provoked chest pains or breathlessness because too little oxygen was supplied to your heart muscle when you exerted yourself. With a slower heart rate and lower blood pressure, your heart muscle would require less oxygen (heart rate and blood pressure largely determine how much oxygen your heart muscle needs). You would, therefore, be less likely to have angina attacks when you exerted yourself, since pain and breathlessness occur when the oxygen needs of the heart muscle exceed the oxygen supply. By lowering the heart rate and blood pressure, you reduce the need of your heart muscle for oxygen, and bring that need into balance with the oxygen supply. But, think of the paradox: in order to achieve slower heart rate and lower blood pressure, you have to exercise regularly and raise your heart rate and blood pressure while doing it!

If a reduction in heart rate and blood pressure is necessary for you because of a heart condition or other reason, there are means other than exercise to achieve these ends. Relatively simple medications are available, and, in fact, are safely and regularly used by millions of people in the United States and around the world. These medications not only lower the heart rate and the blood pessure but also are "cardioprotective," that is, they help to prevent heart attacks. This protective effect has been proved in patients who have already had one heart attack, and many cardiologists believe the protection may extend to those who have not, although no specific studies on this point have been made. So, if a slower heart rate and lower blood pressure are necessary goals because of heart disease, it seems imprudent to undertake a vigorous exercise program to achieve them.

Of course, one can argue that medications have side effects and that it is preferable to achieve things in a "natural" way— as if pushing your body to near exhausting limits and pursuing some arbitrary heart-rate goal are "natural." It's true that medications have side effects. Every medicine may have some side effect in some patients. What is ignored are the possible side

20

effects of exercise—side effects that may be more severe and more dangerous than those due to medications.

In normal individuals, those without cardiovascular disease, one evident change occurs to the heart with prolonged physical training. It is the so-called athlete's heart, where the heart enlarges, at times dramatically. It pumps more blood with each heartbeat and there are microscopic changes of unknown significance within the heart muscle cells. Whether these are biologically beneficial changes is entirely unclear; many of the changes resemble those seen in heart disease. Enlargement of the heart, for example, is often a serious sign of a diseased heart compensating for difficulties in pumping blood—but in an athlete it is said to be a beneficial adaptation to increased performance. Athletes frequently have abnormal electrocardiograms, manifesting changes that in nonathletes would be considered unmistakable signs of disease. The advocates of vigorous exercise training dismiss these as "normal" adaptations. I am not at all sure. Although the athlete's heart may function superiorly, it may not be a healthier heart.

As for increasing maximum oxygen consumption when you are exercising at your peak, there is certainly nothing intrinsically healthier about that. If you're an athlete whose sport requires prolonged exertion and endurance, then it is necessary. If your lifestyle requires the ability to perform more physical work, then you must exercise to achieve that capacity. I have no quarrel with the fact that exercise training is the only way to increase your physical capacity for work. What I do seriously question is the idea that it is healthier.

Fitness is measured physiologically by oxygen consumption, and your body may be efficient in its use of oxygen, so it uses less for a given amount of work performed. But this doesn't mean a thing to your heart, in sickness or in health. People with even severe coronary heart disease can be "trained" with ex-

21

ercise, but it doesn't alter the fact or severity of their coronary artery disease.

Most of the improvement in functional capacity due to exercise is not even directly related to the heart. It is due to an effect on the peripheral muscle cells whereby they more efficiently extract and use oxygen from the blood. Dr. George Sheehan, the "guru" of running, has said, "You might suspect from the emphasis on cardiopulmonary fitness that the major effect of training is on the heart and lungs. Guess again. Exercise does nothing for the lungs; that has been amply proved. . . . Nor does it especially benefit your heart. Running, no matter what you have been told, primarily trains and conditions the muscles."[1]

In people with heart disease especially, virtually all improved fitness is due to changes in the ability of the peripheral muscle cells to extract and use oxygen from the bloodstream. The exact mechanism by which muscle cells become more efficient in removing oxygen and using it to generate and release energy is unknown, but it is not due to any measurable change in the health or the function of the heart. Columbia University cardiologist Dr. Jonathan Moldover denies there is such a thing as "cardiovascular fitness," because fitness is related to peripheral changes.[2]

If physical fitness insured health in general, then only an accident could bring down fit individuals. Certainly if cardiovascular health were either a product or a precondition of physical training, then fit people wouldn't die of heart disease. The fact is that not only do exercisers suffer the usual ills that plague us all, but the leading cause of exercise-related deaths in well-trained people is coronary heart disease.

You can, of course, be fit *and* healthy. Yet you can be physically fit and fatally ill with coronary heart disease, just as you can be wonderfully healthy but quite unfit in terms of exercise capacity. Finally, you can be unfit and unhealthy as well.

It is this last category that poses the greatest problem both to the medical profession and to would-be exercisers. The out-of-shape person who also has atherosclerosis will put quite a strain on a heart already pressed for oxygen in the process of becoming fit. Yet people may undertake exercise without knowing what condition their heart is in, and doctors may prescribe exercise to those they know to have heart disease. Since there is no clear or direct relationship between cardiac health and aerobic fitness, a doctor would like to know *both* how fit a person is and what condition his heart is in before assuring him that he can safely jog two miles a day. Therefore, physicians have sought for ways to diagnose heart disease when it is present, to exclude it when it is absent, and to assess functional capacity. The basic tool in current use is the exercise stress test.

3
What Stress Tests Don't Tell

Each year tens of thousands of newly converted believers are turned loose by physicians to join the millions of already confirmed exercise enthusiasts who pound the streets, fill the parks and line the roadways of our cities and countryside. For thousands more, exercise is formally prescribed and "dosages" established as part of a treatment regimen in the hopes of preventing atherosclerosis, reducing symptoms of angina pectoris or forestalling a heart attack. The approval and the prescription of exercise rest largely on the foundation of a stress test.

The basic concept underlying stress testing is that some abnormalities of the heart that are not apparent when you are at rest may become evident during physical work. Your heart works harder during activity, and performing a physical task—the stress—may provoke abnormal cardiac responses. A stress test thus looks at how the heart performs. How much physical work you can do, of course, depends ultimately on the amount of oxygen your body can use. But oxygen consumption is difficult to measure. Heart rate—the number of heartbeats per minute—is easy to count and record. Since increases in heart rate roughly parallel increases in oxygen consumption during exercise, your heart rate is used as a convenient, although only approximate, measure of how much work you do during the stress test.

If you have consulted a physician within the last few years, the chances are good that a stress test was recommended to you. Perhaps the idea of having a stress test has occurred to you even without a physician's suggestion, since so much is said and written about it. Much of what you hear and see about stress testing is, however, misinformation. Worse, many of those who perform and evaluate the test apparently entertain mistaken and invalid judgments as to its value.

Stress tests are designed mainly to do two things: detect or confirm the presence or absence of heart disease, and establish a safe level of exercise for you. Stress testing does neither of these reliably. It is, in fact, of very limited value and may produce misleading information, sometimes with dangerous consequences.

The various methods of stress testing can be divided into two general categories: single-stage and multistage. In a single-stage test, your level of physical work or stress is kept constant throughout the exercise. The best-known single-stage test is the original Master Two-Step Test, which involves walking up and down two specially constructed steps to increase your oxygen consumption and your heart rate.

The number of times you have to go up and down the steps in a Master Two-Step Test is determined by your age and weight. The older you are, and the heavier, the fewer "trips" over the steps are required. In a single Master Two-Step Test, you make the prescribed number of trips in one and one-half minutes; in the double version, which is preferred by some because it offers a greater total amount of exercise, you make twice the number of trips and do it in twice the length of time. A further refinement is the augmented Double Master Two-Step Test, in which you make an additional number of trips up and down the steps in the same three minutes to increase the work load of your heart.

A less-known, but still occasionally used, single-stage test is the isometric hand-grip test. Here, sustained squeezing with your hands provokes only some increase in heart rate but a significant increase in blood pressure. Rises in blood pressure don't correlate as well with oxygen consumption as increases in heart rate do, so this test is the least valuable one. Since a sudden rise in blood pressure may also have dire consequences for some cardiac patients, this test is generally avoided if you are suspected of having coronary disease.

A multistage test relies on successively increasing levels of activity. You exercise first at a low intensity of effort, and then progressively at higher levels of physical effort. You stay at each level of activity long enough (usually three minutes) for your body to achieve an equilibrium or steady response to that level of activity. Multistage testing can be continuous, going from one level of effort to the next without stopping, or intermittent, with a period of rest after equilibrium at each level of activity is achieved. Most multistage testing today is continuous.

Multistage stress testing is usually done on a treadmill or a stationary exercise bicycle. The differences in results between the two kinds of apparatus are not great, and doctors often decide which to use mostly on the basis of how much they want to spend and how much space they have available. But treadmill testing does have the advantages of using a familiar mode of exercise—namely, walking—and of bringing into use the large muscle groups of the hip and pelvic areas. The treadmill also automatically regulates the work level as long as you continue walking on it.

In treadmill testing you step upon and then walk in time with a moving belt. The level of exercise intensity is varied by the speed and the slope of the treadmill. Tests usually begin with a treadmill speed of 1.7 miles per hour and an upward slope of 10 percent. Successive levels of exercise involve faster speed and steeper slope up to a maximum of 6 miles per hour and a 22 percent grade. Usually, only endurance athletes can perform at this maximum level. Regularly active healthy men can usually complete three minutes of treadmill exercise at 4.2 miles per hour and a 16 percent grade. People who are less fit have, by definition, less capacity for physical work, and their maximum treadmill performance is at lower speeds and grades.

In bicycle testing you sit upon a stationary bicycle. The intensity of the exercise is varied by varying the resistance to pedaling, since the speed of pedaling is kept constant. Unlike the treadmill, where you are forced to carry your own weight and the total amount of oxygen you use for a given amount of effort will therefore vary with your body weight, you are sitting on the bicycle, so the total oxygen requirement for a given amount of pedaling is independent of your body weight. But many people are not accustomed to vigorous bicycle riding; their thigh and calf muscles begin to cramp up or "turn to jelly" before they have hit the peak effort they might be capable of in some other form of exercise.

The end point of a multistage test may vary. Some proponents of stress testing advocate what is called "maximal" testing, which means you exercise to that point where further increase in physical work does not cause further increase in how much oxygen you use or how fast your heart beats. Since heart rate is what is usually measured, maximal exercise for you is that level of effort beyond which your heart rate does not rise any more. At this maximal level, normal people usually feel exhausted, and often nauseated and dizzy as well.

More conservative testers choose a "submaximal" end point for stress testing. In a submaximal test, an arbitrary end point is chosen, usually a heart rate equal to 85 percent of the expected maximum heart rate for your age. Since the expected maximum attainable heart rate decreases as you get older, a convenient formula for predicting average maximum heart rate is 220 minus age. Thus, if you are a normal 40-year-old male having a submaximal exercise test, your predicted maximum attainable heart rate would be 220 minus 40, which equals 180; and 85 percent of that is 153, which represents the arbitrary end point of the test.

If you are a patient with cardiac symptoms, your exercise test is usually symptom-limited. That is, the test is stopped— whatever the level of exercise you achieve—when you report that you are experiencing symptoms of your condition, such as pain, dizziness or breathlessness. Some patients may show signs of abnormal cardiac function, such as pallor or unsteadiness, that can be noted by the examiner even before any symptoms are felt. The test is then stopped at that point, even if the patient still feels comfortable.

Although your performance of the physical effort is the basis of the test, and how you look and feel during the test is important, the examiner relies more on observing and recording your physiologic responses to stress. Many kinds of responses can be measured, including the rate of your heart, its pattern of electrical activity, your blood pressure and oxygen consumption. Whereas all of these responses are measured in a few technically sophisticated testing centers, in most testing situations only the electrical responses of your heart (which automatically give the heart rate) and perhaps your blood pressure are recorded.

The electrical activity of your heart is revealed in your electrocardiogram, a recording of the electric signals that travel through the heart. The heart cannot beat unless the heart muscle is electrically stimulated. Heartbeat is normally regulated by electric signals, generated within the heart itself, that travel through the muscles causing rhythmic, coordinated pumping contractions. The electrocardiogram shows all the electric signals, so it is very easy to count the number of them and thereby know the heart rate. Analyzing more subtle aspects of pattern and contour of the signals as they appear on the electrocardiogram is much trickier. To be honest, we don't even know all the reasons why a normal electrocardiogram taken while a person is resting looks the way it does, and we certainly don't have all the answers as to why certain electrical changes in the heart occur during exercise or stress. Nevertheless, through experience we have learned to recognize many abnormalities and to judge with fair accuracy what conditions they might indicate.

How detailed an electrocardiogram is depends on the complexity of the equipment used. In all recordings, electric signals from your heart are detected by sensing devices called electrodes that are placed on various parts of your body. A simple electrocardiogram system, using very few recording electrodes, may be used on the generally valid assumption that most abnormalities will be detected. More elaborate systems, using many more electrodes, may be employed, however, since it is known that certain abnormal responses may be missed by the simpler system. Whether these abnormalities detected only by the more elaborate recording systems have any clinical significance is still debatable.

Some testers run the electrocardiogram continuously during exercise, while others record only a brief period at the end of each stage of a multistage test. In the single-stage Master Two-Step Test, the electrocardiogram is not made until immediately after you complete the full exercise. Although more information may be obtained from recording during, as well as after, exercise the "extra information" may be misleading and lead to errors in interpretation. The electrocardiogram is also usually made during the rest period after exercise because, as your circulatory system continues to readjust, abnormalities occasionally become evident that were not detected during the actual exercise or in the first minutes of resting. Some of the deaths that occur as a result of stress testing—and deaths do occur—happen in the period following the actual exercise.

Even taking your blood pressure, so simple and standardized a procedure when you're sitting still, becomes a complicated maneuver during stress testing. Blood pressure is the actual pressure of the blood, measured in millimeters of mercury, within the arterial system of the body. With you bobbing up and down, scrambling to keep pace with a treadmill or furiously pedaling a bicycle going nowhere, it is very hard for someone to measure your blood pressure accurately with the standard cuff around your arm. Some testers, therefore, ignore your blood pressure altogether or record it only infrequently during the test. Yet, accurately recorded blood-pressure responses to exercise may be very helpful in diagnosing abnormalities of the heart. In some centers where highly sophisticated physiologic studies are performed, a needle or catheter connected to a sensitive pressure gauge may be inserted directly into one of your arteries for direct measurement of your blood pressure as you exercise.

The results of a test using an elaborate electrocardiogram system may not be reliably compared with results from a simpler one, just as differences in the timing and the method of measuring either electrical or pressure responses give the examiner different data from which to make judgments. Looking at one set of measurements, a doctor might feel that a patient had a perfectly normal heart. Using another set of measurements, he might be just as certain the same heart was abnormal. These differences in testing procedures, techniques and equipment affect the examiner's conclusions about the actual state of an individual's heart.

In spite of these variations in data that can lead to differing interpretations, examiners assume that stress testing does accomplish its basic aims: to diagnose or exclude heart disease and to measure the performance you are capable of. Most people "pass" their stress test. Their cardiac health is certified, they are told what "shape" they're in and they go off to buy their new athletic gear. When the bill arrives, they pay it willingly. It's worth the money to know they're well and that it's safe to exercise. But they *don't* know that, and neither does their doctor. Just as important, when people who "fail" their stress test are told they have heart disease, that conclusion may be equally uncertain.

The most common purpose of stress testing is to find out whether you do or don't have coronary heart disease. That's what the Committee on Exercise of the American Heart Association says,[1] and that's what most doctors think they are doing when they suggest you take a stress test. Many of you considering having a stress test probably have this objective in mind, too—to detect coronary heart disease if it is present. Implied in this is the notion that if the stress test does not reveal coronary heart disease, then you can conclude with confidence that you are free from it.

The trouble is that this conclusion is wrong. A stress test doesn't necessarily detect coronary heart disease, and a normal test is not firm evidence of the absence of coronary disease.

A stress test shows how well you can perform when pushed to work hard during exercise. It is a test of function or performance. But coronary heart disease is structural, a narrowing of the coronary arteries that carry oxygen-laden blood to the heart muscle. It is not a disease of performance, and may not interfere with function at all. You can have nice, clean coronary

31

arteries but a heart that doesn't perform well during hard work. You can have a heart that carries you through a stress test with flying colors but coronary arteries that are already constricted with fatty deposits.

Even if your electrocardiogram and other measures show something unusual in the way you function during a stress test, coronary heart disease is only one of many possible reasons, some of which are innocuous and don't indicate anything one way or another about either the presence of disease or how much exercise you're capable of. In fact, abnormalities in even resting electrocardiograms are not at all uncommon, and are often related to harmless and noncoronary conditions. Many physicians will not do a stress test if your resting electrocardiogram reveals such changes, because it is so likely that the stress test will appear to be abnormal.

Even if your resting electrocardiogram looks perfectly normal, there are many conditions that can make your stress electrocardiogram look abnormal. Abnormalities of heart valves, for example, may be associated with abnormal exercise tests. If you take certain medicines, for another example, the stress electrocardiogram may be abnormal. Anemia, with its low red blood cell count, can produce an abnormal stress test. And high blood pressure, too, may be the cause of abnormal electrocardiogram responses. Yet, with these conditions, exercise would not necessarily be limited or proscribed to the same extent it would be if coronary disease were responsible for the abnormal electrocardiogram.

Sometimes, if you have simply eaten within an hour or two of the stress test, it will look abnormal. This was the case with a prominent business executive who is now chairman of the board of one of the major corporations in the country. His stress test, reviewed at the request of the company underwriting the insurance aspects of his potential appointment, was abnormal.

When the test was repeated after he had had no food for several hours, it was perfectly normal, and a major personal and corporate problem evaporated.

The other side of the coin—the inability of a normal exercise test to exclude the presence of coronary heart disease—is about as common. You can have narrowing of your coronary arteries, even of severe degree, and respond normally to a stress test.

Sometimes the technique of recording the exercise electrocardiogram is inadequate, or the test has been stopped too soon, before abnormal responses have a chance to emerge, but there are many other reasons. An old heart attack might prevent the electrocardiogram signs of current coronary trouble from showing up. Also, the resting electrocardiogram patterns of some people can inhibit abnormal responses to stress. Finally, just as some medicines can produce abnormal stress electrocardiograms in the absence of coronary disease, so can certain medicines prevent an abnormal stress electrocardiogram in the presence of coronary heart disease.

An exercise stress test cannot achieve its major goal of accurately detecting coronary artery disease or ruling it out in any given individual. Although the director of a well-known exercise testing center suggests that it gives "an indirect image of the extent that atherosclerosis has narrowed the individual coronary vessels," exercise testing really gives only very limited and nonspecific information about some cardiovascular responses to one form of stress. Stress testing is definitely an imperfect way to detect or exclude coronary disease, but proponents argue that it might nevertheless be reliable enough. What degree of reliability can you as an individual put on the result of your test?

One way to check a test's reliability is to see how sensitive it is—how often it really picks up coronary heart disease. A perfectly sensitive test would pick up every case of heart disease, and would be 100 percent sensitive. If the test picks up 90 abnormal results out of 100 people with coronary disease the sensitivity is 90 percent. A second way to check a test's reliability is to see how specific it is—how often a normal result really indicates that the person is free of coronary disease. With a perfectly specific test, everyone who showed a normal result would have normal coronary arteries, and the test would be 100 percent specific. If 100 people do not have coronary disease, and 90 of them have a normal test, the specificity of the test is 90 percent.

An abnormal test result is called a "positive" result, meaning something *has* been found. A normal test result is called "negative"—nothing has been found. People who have coronary disease but have a negative test are said to have a "false negative" test. People who do not have coronary disease but have a positive test are said to have a "false positive" test. If 100 people have coronary disease and 90 of them have a positive or abnormal test, and 10 of them have a negative or normal test, then the sensitivity is 90 percent, and the false negative rate is 10 percent. Likewise, if 100 people do not have coronary disease and 90 of them have a negative or normal test, and 10 of them have a positive or abnormal test, the specificity is 90 percent, and the false positive rate is 10 percent.

Many studies have been done to determine the sensitivity, the specificity, the false positive and false negative rates in exercise stress testing. Sensitivity has been estimated as low as about 40 percent and as high as over 90 percent; usually it's considered to be about 75 percent. In other words, the test does pick up 75 percent of people who do have coronary disease. But the remaining 25 percent of the people with coronary disease show nothing unusual in their stress tests, so the false negative rate is 25 percent. In studies that have reported the least sensitivity, the false negative rate is 60 percent, meaning the test misses 60 out of every 100 people who do have coronary disease.

Figures for specificity of stress testing have also varied widely, from as low as 65 percent to as high as 95 percent. If we're to believe the low figure, 65 percent of normal people show a normal electrocardiogram in their stress test, but 35 percent of these healthy men and women, without coronary disease, have a falsely abnormal or false positive test. Reported figures for false positive results—abnormal tests for normal people—range from 5 percent to as high as 35 percent. And in certain special noncoronary subgroups, such as women with a minor heart-valve abnormality and normal coronary arteries, positive tests have been recorded for as many as 64 percent.

This tremendous variability in these test results must, by itself, suggest some real problems, not only with the actual reliability of stress-testing procedures, but also even with how to figure out reliably how reliable they are. Worse, this variability of results *underestimates* the problem of reliability as far as you as an individual are concerned. Most studies of stress testing have involved people known to have, or strongly suspected of having, coronary heart disease. If you test a group of people most of whom probably do have the disease you're testing for, then obviously most of the positive tests will be true positives, since the people do, in fact, have the disease. But if you test a group of people most of whom do not have the disease, then many of the positive tests will be false positives.

If you as an individual know that you have coronary disease, or strongly suspect it, then a stress test adds little or nothing to your knowledge; a positive test would be expected, and a negative test would be highly suspect of being a false negative. If you have no reason to suspect you have coronary disease, then the reliability of a stress test is particularly poor, since a positive test would likely be a false positive; and a negative test, although expected, could not exclude the possibility of coronary disease.

A study from the National Institutes of Health is particularly relevant in this regard.[2] Among 39 subjects who had no symptoms of heart disease but had abnormal stress tests, only 36 percent had significant coronary disease when their arteries were examined by special x-rays after dye injections directly into the coronary circulation. The results in 64 percent of their positive or abnormal stress tests were simply wrong for the diagnosis of significant coronary artery disease. A similar study by the United States Air Force found 75 percent false positive stress tests in people without symptoms who nevertheless underwent exercise testing.[3]

Stress testing in women is especially misleading, for reasons that are not the least bit clear. In some studies, more than half the positive stress tests for coronary disease in women are false positive, indicating disease where none exists. Women might as well toss a coin to see whether or not they have coronary disease as rely on the results of a traditional stress test.

Another measure of a test's reliability is its reproducibility— how often results come out the same when the test is repeated. To consider a test a reliable indicator of anything, you should expect that repeating the test under the same conditions will give results that are very similar, if not identical, each time. Imagine an IQ test in which you got a score of 80 one day and 150 the next. Since intelligence doesn't vary much from day to day—and neither does the condition of arteries—test results that fluctuate that way have no meaning. A measure of something must be reproducible, or else its validity as a standard or measure is compromised.

When the question of reproducibility of stress testing has been addressed, the results are dismaying.

Analyzing the occurrence of irregularities of the heart rhythm during exercise testing shows that reproducibility in two consecutive tests in the same individual is about equal to reproducibility by chance alone.[4] If you test the same group of people repeatedly, different members of the group will have arrhythmias on each test. Tests done as close as 45 minutes apart and those done months and years apart show the same lack of reproducibility.[5]

Perhaps the most telling report was delivered at the scientific sessions of the American College of Cardiology in 1977.[6] The purpose of the study was to assess the reproducibility of the most abnormal stress tests, the tests that suggested the most severe degree of coronary disease. Of 34 subjects who had at least one severely abnormal test, only 14 had reproducibly abnormal stress tests, while for the 20 other people the severely abnormal response could not be reproduced. And in 11 of these 20 who did not have reproducible tests, at least one of the repeat tests was actually normal. Thus, only 41 percent of markedly abnormal stress tests were reproducible, and 59 percent were not.

Much as any doctor—and that includes me—would appreciate a foolproof way to check easily for coronary disease, stress tests are not sensitive enough, specific enough or reproducible enough for anyone to be sure they're telling you anything at all. At most, a stress test might have some value in confirming a diagnosis already arrived at by the conventional means of carefully taking a patient's medical history.

The best analysis of whether a stress test provides usable additional information for you or your physician comes from Victor Froelicher, formerly of the United States Air Force School of Aerospace Medicine and now with the University of California, San Diego.[7] Dr. Froelicher summarized several previous studies of the accuracy of diagnosing coronary heart disease just from the patient's history—the symptoms the patient related to his physician. Diagnosis of the presence of coronary disease was accurate 90 percent of the time from symptoms alone. In patients with no symptoms like those of coronary disease, the diagnosis of absence of coronary disease was correct in 95 percent of the cases, while in 5 percent there was latent or hidden coronary disease.

Dr. Froelicher then calculated, based on average sensitivity, specificity and reliability figures, how much more certainty could be achieved if a stress test were done. He concluded that a positive or abnormal stress test for a patient already thought to have coronary disease through symptoms alone raised the probability of the diagnosis being correct from 90 percent to 98 percent. A negative or normal stress test in a patient thought to have coronary disease lowered the probability of the diagnosis being correct from 90 percent to 75 percent.

In patients with no symptoms at all, a positive or abnormal stress test raised the probability of hidden coronary disease from 5 percent to 27 percent, while a negative or normal stress test reduced the probability of coronary disease from 5 percent to 2 percent.

At first glance, the changes in probability of having coronary disease based on results of stress testing might look significant and, to an epidemiologist concerned with huge groups of people, they probably are. But think about yourself as an individual. Since there are so many false positive and false negative tests, no individual can tell if his or her own test is a true positive or true negative or false positive or false negative.

If you have a history that indicates coronary heart disease, you already know the probability of your really having coronary disease is 90 percent. A positive stress test that raises the probability to 98 percent doesn't really change anything. And a negative stress test only means that the likelihood of really having coronary disease is somewhat less, but it is still 75 percent. In either case, you'd probably play it safe and conduct your life on the assumption that you're likely to have coronary disease.

By the same token, if you have no history at all indicating

coronary disease, and the probability of really not having coronary disease is about 95 percent, an abnormal stress test only means the probability of not having coronary disease is somewhat reduced, but it is still 75 percent. In other words, the chances are still three out of four that you're quite well and needn't worry about having coronary disease, because the test is likely to have been a false positive.

On the basis of your medical history alone, an accurate enough estimate of the likelihood that you have coronary disease can be made. A stress test does not offer significant additional information—it may offer only additional confusion—and is therefore quite unnecessary.

But let us assume you undergo a stress test. A positive or abnormal test is obviously of greater concern than a negative or normal one. So, let's assume the results are abnormal.

You are now faced with the question of whether the abnormal test is a true positive or a false positive one.

You have a few options in this circumstance, but none are very satisfactory. First, you may decide to ignore the test result and rely on the information you had about yourself before the test. If this is your choice, why did you spend your time and money to have the test in the first place? And you may be left, as many people are, with a nagging sense of anxiety about the underlying condition of your heart.

A second choice is to have a repeat stress test. Whoever conducted your first test would probably willingly do another. After all, it's your time and your money. But reproducibility is so poor that you'll be stuck with essentially the same problem after the repeat test. If the repeat is positive, is it a true positive or a false positive? If it is negative this time, which test was correct, the first or the second? No matter how many tests you undergo, their reliability is questionable.

Further choices in following up abnormal stress tests are

radionuclide scanning and coronary angiography. The first involves injecting radioactive material into the bloodstream and following its course through the heart or coronary circulation. Accuracy of some forms of scanning is not much better than that of regular stress testing. Newer scanning techniques are more accurate but the cost may be over $500. Angiography usually requires hospitalization, because tubes are inserted directly into the heart and coronary arteries. Death and serious nonfatal complications occur in a small percentage of patients.

Besides the detection or exclusion of coronary heart disease—which it fails to achieve reliably—the other major aim of exercise testing is to find your exercise capacity and what level of exercise is safe for you. The Committee on Exercise of the American Heart Association advises that "exercise intensity that is both safe and effective must be based on the individual's exercise tolerance or capacity . . . a measurement or accurate estimate of individual tolerance . . . is an extremely useful aid to choosing the proper intensity at the beginning of an exercise program." The committee adds that "exercise intensity must be regulated periodically during the succeeding stages" of an exercise program.[8]

In their exercise handbook for physicians, the Heart Association also says that "individuals who complete testing without exhibiting abnormal ECG [electrocardiogram] responses or other evidence of overt or subclinical heart disease can be medically authorized to take part in unsupervised exercise of an intensity that does not exceed that achieved during the clearance test." In other words, according to this, if you once complete a maximal stress test to the level of exercise where your heart rate and oxygen usage cannot increase further despite more exercise, and you don't show abnormal responses, then you can feel safe in pushing yourself to that level regularly. If your test is a submaximal one, say, to 85 percent of your age-predicted maximum heart rate, then this level of exercise may be regularly performed with impunity.

This is a splendid ideal—the accurate estimation of your individual tolerance for stress, and the periodic adjustment of your activity to your changing capacity. Unfortunately, it is an elusive one. I fully subscribe to the ideal, but I dispute the Committee on Exercise when it implies that even the most sophisticated, monitored, multistage exercise testing can achieve it.

If you accept that stress testing gives an accurate estimate of your tolerance or capacity for physical exercise, you're assuming that your exercise capacity is fixed and stable. But that isn't so. There are lots of things that can change your responses to the same amount of physical stress. Some of these things are under your direct control: smoking, eating, drinking. Other things, perhaps beyond your control, are equally important: temperature, humidity, air quality, worry, anger, depression. All of these can significantly affect your cardiovascular responses and your general body reactions to running, cycling, aerobic dancing—whatever kind of vigorous exercise you like to do.

It's naive to assume that you'll always respond to exercise the same way you did in the controlled environment of your stress test. You can't run in 90° heat the way you can in an air-conditioned office. You can't play squash as well if you've just polished off a pound of lasagna. And cigarettes have got to slow you down on the tennis court.

The vogue today is for physicians to "prescribe" exercise, especially for cardiac patients, much as they prescribe medications, with specific "dosages" based on stress-test performance. This lends an unwarranted air of scientific precision to stress testing and adds to the credibility of the erroneous idea that exercise is medically beneficial. But it doesn't alter the fact

41

that your cardiac and other responses to a specific amount of physical activity vary with circumstances. These responses may be entirely and dangerously unpredictable.

A tragic true story illustrates the point. A twenty-seven-year-old man who exercised regularly and repeatedly underwent maximal stress tests with normal results suffered cardiac arrest running on a track where he had run often for years. He never exceeded the level of exercise that he easily achieved in stress testing. We learned later that he had had several drinks the night before and had slept poorly following an argument with his estranged wife. His response to exercise on that fateful day was not predicted or even suspected by any test he had ever had. Nobody ever tested him under his "real-life" conditions, nor is it possible to do so.

Actually, stress testing itself carries risks. You'll note that you're asked to sign a release form before a test, indication enough of at least some potential danger. The largest study of risks associated with stress testing in the United States appeared in the *Journal of the American Medical Association* in 1971, and indicated 1 death per 10,000 tests in a survey of 170,000 tests performed at various centers around the country.[9] When serious nonfatal complications were included, the incidence rose to 2.5 morbid events per 10,000 tests. A larger and more recent study from West Germany reported 1 complication in every 7,500 exercise stress tests.[10] Using the 1 in 7,500 figures, if just the estimated 30 million joggers in the United States each had 1 stress test yearly, we could anticipate 4,000 such dangerous incidents. A more recent American study covering 1,375 centers showed 8.86 complications per 10,000 tests;[11] one of the authors of that study reported 3 deaths in his own series of 10,000 tests.[12]

In all likelihood, the figures are but the tip of the iceberg and underestimate the dangers because many untoward events and complications are not publicly reported. Also, many stress tests are probably performed where preparation and supervision are not optimal, and statistics from such testing sites are likely to be worse but to go unreported. More tragic, a significant number of the reported deaths and life-threatening complications occur to people whose coronary arteries are subsequently shown to be normal.

If you still assume that stress testing gives an accurate estimate of how hard you can safely exercise, then it's only logical that you be willing to spend your time and money, and take the risk, of periodically updating your stress test. Exercise capacity can diminish as well as increase due to a variety of causes, including illness and inactivity. It takes just a short time—a few days to a few weeks at most—to lose most or all of the conditioning benefits of physical training, and you should be willing to be retested after any significant interruption of your exercise routine and periodically during any exercise program—at $150 or more a shot.

Of course, few people undergo regularly repeated stress testing; why should they when they hear from all sides that exercise itself will prevent the very disease that the test is supposed to detect? Armed with assurance that they do not have coronary artery disease, most patients leave the ordeal of their first stress test to embrace wholeheartedly what they believe to be the protection of exercise.

4
The Case against Longevity

Longevity is the most compelling of the promised protections of exercise. Millions of today's exercise enthusiasts, seduced into the latest warm-up gear, designer labels sticking to their sweating bodies, run, dance, stretch and strain in the hope and expectation of living longer lives. But despite the widespread notion that physical exercise can add years to your life, there is no reliable evidence to prove it.

Biological aging is a fact of life. Although some researchers conclude that we have a biological potential of up to 110 or 120 years, living that long is so rare that most scientists settle for a biological limit of about 80 years, barring extraordinary new and fundamental discoveries about the human organism and the aging process itself.

We think of ourselves as living longer than our forebears, but in fact the biological limit hasn't changed. Tombstones in eighteenth- and nineteenth-century cemeteries are witness to the frequency then of infant and childhood mortality, deaths in epidemics and death in childbirth. But the ages of those who did reach "old age" are not different from ages today. Advances in medicine and public health have primarily extended the *average* life expectancy by allowing more people to reach the upper limit of their biological potential. A larger proportion of the population reaches old age these days, but the upper limit of life expectancy has not been dramatically altered. If the two leading causes of death today—cardiovascular disease and cancer—were conquered, overall life expectancy would still increase by only a few years.

Given the biological limit to longevity, the likelihood of attaining that age depends upon many things. Diseases, although different ones from those that took our forebears to early graves, are still important. But other, less tangible, circumstances, generally lumped under the label "psychosocial variables," seem to matter as much, since they affect mortality to a large degree. For example, at any given age more than twice as many people from the "lowest" social class die as from the "highest" social class. And men with less than eight years of schooling have a 50 percent higher death rate than those completing one or more years of college.[1]

Because psychosocial variables can exert a large influence on any analysis of mortality, a valid study of the relationship between physical activity and longevity must take a long list of them into account. Studies that don't—and that is nearly all of them—are simplistic and unreliable.

Besides social group and educational status, the best-documented psychosocial variables that influence longevity are income, occupational status, work satisfaction, social activity and life satisfaction. People who are more prosperous, who hold higher-level positions, who find their work and their social lives interesting and gratifying live longer!

Social interaction seems to be one of the most important predictors of longevity. Men and women with the most social connections live longest, while those whose lifestyles isolate them from other people are more likely to die sooner. The elderly church volunteer who bustles about at the church bazaar is likely to be living longer because she is socially active, not because she is physically so. Married people live longer than the unmarried, the widowed and the divorced. Even pets may provide a form of social interaction; people with pets live longer, too.

An underlying reason may be that pleasant social interactions tend to reduce stress. Stress has been glaringly implicated as an unhealthy ingredient in our lives. Although a few people seem to thrive on stress, and a moderate amount of pressure may have some beneficial effect, larger dosages for most people can produce destructive changes in their bodies' hormone and other chemical balances. These changes may, in turn, affect susceptibility to disease or hamper the ability to fight off disease once it occurs. The first year of retirement and the first year of widowhood—hard times for all of us—are both associated with a jump in mortality rates. Even the surprising parallel of higher death rates with unemployment probably has its origin in tension-related illness and physiological vulnerability. A study of 1,200 centenarians, Americans from farmers to bankers who lived to be at least one hundred years old, showed absence of stress, for whatever reason, to be the most fundamental common denominator in their long lives.[2]

Heredity, nutrition, habits and environment are other factors that affect the length of our lives. If your parents, your Great-Aunt Matilda and your Grandfather Jones all lived to be ninety, you can make a fair guess that longevity "runs in the family." What you eat and whether you smoke or drink alcohol in more than moderate amounts affect health in general, and therefore longevity. Mortality rates vary by where a person lives, partly because of such factors as industrial pollution, but also because of such measures as the pace of life, the social integration possible and the extent of community support systems of all kinds.

Clearly, the issue of longevity is enormously complex. So many things—many of which are poorly understood and very difficult to measure—are involved that predicting the life span of any individual is virtually impossible. If marriage itself is protective, does a "bad" marriage work just as well? And if not, how happy must the marriage be, and how do you measure that? A person might be delighted with his job as a coal miner, but easily contract "black lung" in his forties. Mrs. Smith might volunteer for every committee in sight out of strident contempt for the incompetence of her co-workers, so that the fact of her membership is a poor measure of her social interaction.

Into this morass of ill-defined and unquantifiable elements has been dropped the complicated question of exercise and *its* relationship to longevity. However ill-founded, the idea that exercise is protective and life-enhancing is compelling. Children, who can run about all day, strike us as "full of life," and we say of an active older person that she is "brimming with vitality." When we are full of life, it often brims over in the form of activity. What is more logical, then, than to build from this the notion that exercise *puts* more life into a person? The idea is accepted by most people as a biological "given." There is an almost unassailable belief that exercise adds more life, and that we will therefore not die so early. The idea has a simple and intuitive logic, a seductive, magical quality.

Studies of the relationship between physical activity and mortality deal almost exclusively with death from coronary disease, and with good reason. Cardiovascular disease is the leading cause of death in industrialized societies, and any measurable impact on life expectancy would have to affect a major cause of death. Physical activity is, moreover, dependent upon the cardiovascular system at least to the extent that the heart pumps the blood and the arteries carry it around the body so the cells can use the oxygen in it to provide energy for activity. No one has even suggested a link between physical activity and other major causes of death, such as cancer or car accidents.

Research in this area is thoroughly confused. In study after study of physical activity and mortality, results are so contradictory that any conclusion that could be drawn from them amounts to no more than unsubstantiated opinion.

The specific belief that exercise makes you live longer because it protects you from coronary disease was first legitimized by Jeremy Morris's 1953 landmark study of London transport workers. Morris analyzed the health records of about 31,000 male London transport workers, ages thirty-five to sixty-four years, in order to "seek for relations between the kind of work men do . . . and the incidence among them of coronary heart-disease." The workers were divided into two occupational work groups, conductors and drivers. London bus conductors are a pretty active group; they swing up and down the stairs of the double-deckers, help little old ladies on, rush to tell people where to get off and manage to collect all the fares in the meantime; the drivers, on the other hand, just sit behind the wheel and drive. The results of the data analysis showed that conductors had less coronary heart disease than the drivers; when the disease did appear in conductors, it was at a later age and was less severe; and conductors lived longer. Morris and his colleagues focused on the greater physical activity of "conducting" to explain the lower incidence and mortality of coronary heart disease.

Physicians quickly accepted these conclusions as scientific fact. The impact was such that most subsequent studies of the relationship between activity and coronary disease and longevity, even to this day, cite Morris's original study as a foundation. The force of the "facts" was so great that, although Morris and his co-workers repudiated their original conclusions within only three years—we shall see why—others still sought to confirm what had never been proven in the first place. Support for the idea that physical activity enhanced longevity and reduced coronary heart disease appeared regularly in medical journals during the 1960s. By the following decade, the medical profession was, literally, off to the races.

In 1962, H. L. Taylor, of the University of Minnesota School of Public Health, analyzed records of 191,609 men employed in the American railroad industry, an industry chosen because it offered "favorable conditions for study."[3] Railroad workers rarely change jobs, so the effects of other occupational influences are minimized. Since detailed records are usually maintained, data on death rates are considered reliable. Taylor's analysis showed lower death rates for more active people, supporting the idea that men in sedentary occupations have more coronary heart disease than those whose work requires moderate to heavy physical activity.

An analysis of about 110,000 adults enrolled in the Health Insurance Plan of Greater New York, and classified by activity levels, was published in 1969.[4] The least active group had twice the risk (8.5 per 1,000 compared with 4.2 per 1,000) of suffering a first heart attack compared with the next active group; and dying from that heart attack was also more likely for the least active individuals. The differences were only between sedentary men and those moderately more active. There was no further decrease in risk for more active people.

In 1975, Dr. Ralph S. Paffenberger, Jr., of Stanford University School of Medicine, analyzed the health records of 6,351 San Francisco–area longshoremen.[5] Trying to correlate work energy expenditure with coronary attacks and coronary deaths, he found that only those longshoremen leading a very energetic work life had significant protection from coronary attacks; lesser degrees of energy expenditure were not protective.

Dr. Paffenberger later analyzed 16,936 questionnaires of supposedly healthy Harvard alumni who had entered the school from 1916 to 1950.[6] He estimated energy expenditure from the activities the respondents reported—everything from reading to squash, from doing nothing to distance running and competitive team games. The data reportedly indicated that high-level energy expenditure was protective against fatal and non-fatal coronary heart disease, but anything less than high-level energy expenditure was of little or no protective value.

About 20 years after Morris's appealing findings, the popularity of running began really catching on. Since the 1972 Olympic Games, when millions of television viewers saw Frank Shorter become the first American in 64 years to win the marathon, interest and involvement with running grew. The New York Road Runners Club, which had started in 1958 with 42 members, had, by 1976, some 1,700 members; it now numbers about 22,000. The 1970 New York Marathon attracted only 126 runners, and almost five times that number ten years later. In 1975, the New York Road Runners Club began classes and clinics to promote and provide instruction in running. A highly successful magazine, *The Runner*, began publication in 1978, and three books on running were on the *New York Times* best-seller list for much of that same year.

In the running glory days of the 1970s, a quite extraordinary idea was introduced to the medical profession and then, rather quickly, to the running world at large. Popularly known as the "Marathon Hypothesis," the notion was formulated by Dr. Thomas J. Bassler, a pathologist in California. As originally proposed by Dr. Bassler, himself a devoted marathoner, the thesis stated that marathon running conferred absolute protection against death from coronary heart disease.[7]

During the ensuing years, the Marathon Hypothesis was quoted and misquoted, defined and redefined, as various people used it to support or deny one or another proposition. The resulting confusion arises partly from the fact that Dr. Bassler himself has restated the idea repeatedly, but with different words and with different emphasis. Originally, the proposition seemed to be that marathon running itself protects one from death due to coronary heart disease. More recently, Dr. Bassler's focus has changed; he now credits the lifestyle of the marathon runner, rather than the running itself, with conferring this remarkable immunity. According to him, any person whose lifestyle permits him to complete a 42-kilometer race—a traditional marathon— is immune to dying from coronary artery disease. Others have taken the proposition even farther afield. Believe it or not, even the notion of immortality as a consequence of marathon running has been suggested.

Thus, with Morris's original publication in 1953, the subsequent apparent confirmations during the 1960s and 1970s, and the dramatic impact of the Marathon Hypothesis a decade ago, the idea that physical activity is life-enhancing was firmly established. The case for longevity had come a long way.

Intuitively appealing ideas that have both logical and magical qualities perhaps are too difficult to dispel. But it still seems odd in retrospect that these studies and ideas were not subjected to a more critical eye and that more credence was not given to similar studies that failed to show a connection between physical activity and longevity, or even showed that a strenuous life could lead to an earlier death.

Maybe the enthusiasm generated by Morris's original study was too great to suggest a more critical appraisal. After all, if physical activity could reduce the incidence and severity of what was becoming recognized as an epidemic of coronary heart disease, it was within the power of each of us to prevent this epidemic from spreading to those we cared for and to ourselves. This easy answer—be more active—was too appealing to generate sufficient controversy and conflict.

But there were reasons enough to question the validity of the conclusions that the exercise enthusiasts had reached, if only anyone had wanted to.

From the beginning, Morris and his colleagues listed other possible explanations for their bus driver and conductor data and were quite honest in announcing their bias. They chose to focus on the "greater physical activity of conducting" as the cause of the lower incidence of coronary heart disease and mortality in that group, and "decided to ignore . . . the other factors in the constitution of the men and in their history that must certainly also be involved." These "other factors" they listed but chose to ignore included: "differences in the constitution and early experience of the conductors and drivers, another expression of which is that the men select for themselves these very different jobs."

These "differences in the constitution" and the consequent self-selection of different jobs by different people are, in fact, central to a critical analysis of Morris's data. For, as he himself found and published in 1956, only three years after his original report, the conductors and drivers were really not similar people from the outset.[8] The bus drivers were fatter; their girth and weight were greater than that of conductors even at the time they were first hired. And if being fatter went along with things like higher cholesterol levels and blood pressure, as seems likely, then these could have explained the differences in the risk of dying observed later.

This self-selection of certain occupations and activities by people who already have certain characteristics that affect longevity is a problem that plagues all such studies. It confounds the analysis of the relationship of activity itself to longevity, since these other characteristics have already influenced the choice of activity. That this was not a fluke or an isolated aberration of Morris's study was shown by a report in 1967 by R. M. Oliver, of Great Britain, who studied the physiques and levels of blood fats of recruits for the jobs of bus conductor and bus driver in London before the activity of the job itself could affect the men.[9] He concluded: "It is apparent that British men with certain physical characteristics choose or are chosen to become bus drivers as opposed to conductors," and added that his study "supports the view that inherited characteristics, one of which may be susceptibility to heart disease, may predispose to a particular occupation."

This self-selection of activity by virtue of inherited or other preexisting characteristics affects studies relating any type of activity, occupational or recreational, to health and longevity. The fathers of marathon runners, for example, have less coronary heart disease than the fathers of individuals who are not marathoners. Since those who choose to run marathons have less inherited family history of coronary disease than do nonmarathoners, this already makes those 42-kilometer men less prone to coronary disease and mortality, even if they never even ran to catch a bus.

Similar self-selection operates in the area of blood cholesterol levels. Although reports indicate, for example, that running favorably affects cholesterol levels for cardiovascular health, it's also true that even before they begin to run, individuals who choose to become runners already have better cholesterol levels than those who choose not to run. People with certain preexisting characteristics or qualities select certain activities and lifestyles, although we don't know why. It is these preexisting characteristics, rather than the activity that they seem to lead to, that may be beneficial.

In Taylor's 1962 study of American railroad-industry employees, other problems affected the validity of his conclusions. Lower death rates in more active people turned up only in workers of certain age groups. For instance, only among sixty- to sixty-four-year-olds were overall deaths more common in the most inactive than in moderately active workers. For all other age groups, overall death rates were similar. When the most inactive were compared with the most active, overall deaths were lower only among active workers aged fifty-five to fifty-nine and sixty to sixty-four. For deaths due solely to coronary heart disease, the least active men had higher mortality rates compared with moderately active men in age groups forty to forty-four, fifty-five to fifty-nine and sixty to sixty-four, but death rates were similar for ages forty-five to forty-nine and fifty to fifty-four. And comparing coronary deaths of the least active with the most active workers, death rates for the least active were higher for ages forty-five to forty-nine, fifty-five to fifty-nine and sixty to sixty-four, but were not different for the ages of forty to forty-four and fifty to fifty-four. Since there is no logical or biological reason for these figures, chance or something else completely unrelated to physical activity seems the more likely explanation. Furthermore, there are no data to indicate that these railroad employees were really representative of the rest of the population. For all we know, and as Taylor himself suggested, they may have been a unique group, with many characteristics not shared by the rest of us. Perhaps most important, more of the sedentary workers lived in urban centers, where death rates are higher anyway, and the most active group were apt to live in small communities, where death rates are generally lower. This alone can invalidate the conclusion that the level of physical activity caused the observed differences in mortality rates among the different workers.

In the 1969 Health Insurance Plan study, data were obtained by reviewing the medical records of 110,000 people enrolled in the health plan. Most of those who met the criteria for coronary heart disease were specially examined and interviewed. To determine the characteristics, including physical activity, of the population, a random 12 percent of the entire 110,000 people received a questionnaire during the three years of the study, but only 83 percent responded. Only 156 patients had a special examination *and* an interview *and* answered the mail survey questionnaire. How people described their activity levels when probed by an interviewer didn't correspond well with what they had filled out on the mailed form, forcing the study's authors themselves to advise considerable caution in interpreting the findings. Also, other variables, including cholesterol levels and psychosocial factors that might have influenced the risk associated with physical inactivity, weren't even considered, and these and other unidentified factors might have independently contributed to both inactivity and heart attacks.

The longshoremen study in 1975 conspicuously ignored the bias of job self-selection, which the London transport workers study had showed to be so important. Also, because it was possible that men had recently changed jobs due to poor health, deaths were related to the jobs held six months before they died. But it seems most plausible to me that the onset of symptoms of coronary heart disease would usually come more than six months before death. So people who may have been very active when their heart disease began were listed as inactive when they died.

The longshoremen's union regulations divide each working hour of the heavy-work group into 55 percent work and 45 percent rest, and for the light-work group, 75 percent of each hour is devoted to work and only 25 percent to rest. While the authors credit the "repeated bursts of peak effort" for the lower coronary risk among heavy workers, I find it deliciously appealing to credit their longer rest periods. Certainly the study failed to consider factors such as lack of job satisfaction, less conviviality, even the sheer boredom that sedentary work might have entailed.

If Dr. Paffenburger's longshoremen study was flawed, so was his later Harvard alumni study. For some reason, those who answered the questionnaire were considerably healthier than alumni who failed to respond. The fact that those who did respond weren't representative of Harvard alumni in general was easy to tell: Harvard keeps records of all alumni deaths, and as the years passed it turned out that those who had responded to the survey weren't dying off as fast as those who hadn't. That should teach us a lesson in statistics. If you want to live longer, the numbers seem to say, answer a Harvard alumni questionnaire.

In depending on questionnaire information about physical activity, the study relied on a mail survey, a method the Health Insurance Plan study and others have shown to be unreliable. The questionnaire, anyway, failed to include questions about personality, stress, levels of blood fat and other factors likely to be important in coronary disease and overall longevity. Moreover, about one out of five respondents who claimed to have no heart disease actually did have coronary heart disease. It seems logical that those who had heart disease, whether they were unaware of it or simply preferred not to report it, would nevertheless have lower activity levels, either because of symptom limitation such as pain, breathlessness or dizziness, or because of those subtle and still-unidentified factors that make sick people do less. These Harvard men would have an increased mortality rate due to their preexisting heart disease, but in the study it would be attributed to their inactivity.

All this picking away at studies that imply that you can live longer if you exercise might seem trivial if all the studies around came to the same conclusion. But many investigations show no difference at all in death rates of muscled, sinewy, outdoorsy types compared with sedentary desk workers. There are even studies demonstrating earlier death for more active people.

A 1970 study of Italian railroad men showed that neither overall death rate nor coronary heart disease death rate was related to occupational physical activity.[10] Another look at United States railroad men indicated that death rates from *all causes* were *higher* among physically active switchmen than men in sedentary occupations even though the coronary death rate was lower among the more active men. And what differences there were were those you might find by chance alone. A seven-country study concluded that if levels of physical activity or inactivity were related to coronary heart disease, it was such a minor association that it probably couldn't even be proven.[11]

Six years later, an analysis of 172,459 Italian railroad workers also found overall death rates from all causes higher among men performing heavy work compared with moderate and sedentary workers.[12] Again, sedentary people had increased mortality from coronary heart disease, but the heavy-work group died sooner of "degenerative heart disease," a catchall term that includes many cases of coronary heart disease.

Dr. John M. Chapman and his colleagues found, in a 1957 study of 2,252 Los Angeles civil service employees, 30 percent *fewer* new cases of coronary heart disease than expected based on age in a sedentary group of workers, and 38 percent *more* cases than expected in a heavy-exertion group.[13] Overall, there were 25 percent more new cases of coronary heart disease and deaths from coronary disease in the two highest levels of physical activity compared with the two lowest.

A 1967 analysis of Indian railway workers in the *British Heart Journal* reported that "an unexpected and extraordinary finding in our data is that mortality in the sedentary occupation of clerks is lower than the physically active occupation of fitters . . . this is contrary to the current conceptions of the protective role of exercise."[14] Heavier levels of physical activity conferred no evident protection or benefit; the higher levels of activity were associated with the greatest death rates.

In a Scandinavian study in 1976 comparing several levels of activity of Finnish men, total mortality was *highest* for men doing the most vigorous physical activity.[15] Coronary heart disease mortality didn't generally correlate well with habitual physical exertion, but was clearly highest for the most active men. The authors, members of the Finnish Heart Association, offered the possibility "that vigorous habitual physical activity which exceeds a certain threshold is deleterious or, at least, does not further reduce the risk of coronary heart disease."

No doubt these studies could also be picked apart to reveal their flaws. All such rather unsophisticated uses of statistics are powerless to explain so complicated a thing as why one person dies of a heart attack at fifty, and his neighbor lives on to be one hundred. Studies that claim that physical activity confers longevity are inevitably faulty in design, and just as much contradictory data can be accumulated by the same methods. Jeremy Morris, who maintained his belief that physical activity protected against coronary heart disease, was nevertheless a candid man. "The evidence on this problem is quite conflicting," he admitted. "In several studies coronary heart disease has been found to be associated with physical activity/inactivity in the expected way. In as many, no relationship was demonstrated, or an equivocal or opposite one; and why this is so is still quite unclear."[16]

There is one simple explanation of why the relationship between activity and longevity is unclear. They may not be related. How much you exercise and how long you live may not be connected at all.

If you start with the belief that exercise is beneficial to life, then contrary or conflicting data will certainly be troubling and puzzling. But if you start with no particular assumption, if you approach the subject with an open mind, suddenly there is no problem. Some people who exercise live a long time, some don't; some sedentary people die young, others live to their biological limit. There is about the same relationship between activity and longevity as you might find if you were to compare the amount of chocolate pudding children eat with the likelihood of their coming down with chicken pox—that is, no relationship at all. That's the most reasonable interpretation of the "conflicting" results from all the studies.

Unfortunately, little reason has lit this murky subject. If Morris's London transit worker study had shown either no protection from exercise or actual deleterious effects, as later studies did, then the dilemma of today would not exist. The burden of proof would be on those trying to establish a protective effect of exercise, something they in all likelihood couldn't do. Instead, however, the protective effect of exercise is widely accepted as a biological fact, and the burden of proof falls on those, like me, who doubt it.

Faulting the methodology of studies that purport to show life-extending benefits of exercise and laying out an equal array of data contradicting that notion is still not enough to dispel the ingrained idea that exercise must somehow be good. The exercise believers have a fall-back position: Since coronary disease is an insidious affair, usually unfelt and undiagnosed until it is well advanced, perhaps exercise cannot really undo it once it is well established. But maybe exercise can affect its course, delay its appearance, retard its progression. Perhaps exercise benefits us in a less obvious but nevertheless important way. If we could just find, for example, that exercise did something to the way fats pile up in our arteries, or to the way our arteries respond to damage, or to anything else we know contributes to coronary artery disease, we might then still have a treatment we should respect and recommend.

5

The Inside Evidence

Exercise enthusiasts may well object to having their claims to longevity dispelled by attacks on numbers and methods, and by citing contradictory studies done in the same manner. Statistics are tricky, and hard enough for epidemiologists to handle. What about the effects of exercise on things that lead to heart trouble, and what about the physical evidence, the actual hearts and arteries of those who exercise and those who don't?

Scientists and researchers have sometimes tried to look at exercise as it might affect the heart at different stages in the development of cardiovascular disease. There is a certain logic to this, for it could be that exercise might have different effects on your cardiovascular system at different times in your life. Perhaps if started early enough, some people reason, vigorous activity could prevent or forestall the development of atherosclerosis, the accumulation of fatty deposits in the arteries. Others say that if such "primary prevention" does not occur, then exercising after coronary disease has developed might provide "secondary prevention" by slowing up the progress of the disease and minimizing its consequences. Some cardiovascular researchers further refine that thesis, and consider secondary prevention to be prevention at the stage of early vascular disease, before there are any symptoms or signs of it, and "tertiary prevention" to be prevention after there is clinical evidence of disease, such as angina pectoris or a heart attack.

As far as primary prevention goes, there is no good evidence that relates physical activity or the lack of it in early life to the development of coronary atherosclerosis. Autopsies of young American soldiers killed in the Korean and Vietnam wars have shown a surprisingly and disquietingly high incidence of early atherosclerosis. Yet surely most soldiers, tested, trained and forced by circumstance to maintain strenuous levels of exertion, are physically active youths. Judging by arteries alone, however, there was no clue that such a life had any inhibiting effect on the early stages of coronary disease. Going back even further, to activity levels during childhood, Dr. G. R. Osborn, a British pathologist at the University of Sheffield, has studied the coronary arteries of infants and young children killed by traumatic and other noncardiac causes.[1] After years of painstaking and meticulous work on the arteries of over 1,000 subjects (some adult), Dr. Osborn has identified microscopic injuries to the artery walls in infancy that he believes to be the origins of atherosclerotic disease. These injuries have nothing to do with the levels of physical activity of infants and children.

Another way, perhaps, of looking at possible primary prevention of atherosclerosis by exercise is to look at the effects of lack of exercise. Can one at least guess that there are benefits from activity by showing that inactivity leads to coronary heart disease? There is perhaps a hint that inactivity is related to coronary atherosclerosis. But by all indications, you must be truly sedentary—a slug who sits or lies about all day, or barely

crawls from bed to breakfast, to car and desk and back again—
to be at any risk from inactivity. No one who has to push a
vacuum cleaner, play ball with the children or keep the lawn
mowed is that inactive.

Since the evidence for preventing the early stages of coronary heart disease by exercising is virtually nonexistent, what
about secondary and tertiary prevention? Can exercise slow
down the progress of atherosclerosis once it has started or prevent more heart attacks once you have had one? Can exercise
prevent the arrhythmia that causes the sudden cardiac death of
people with coronary heart disease?

These are crucial questions because exercise programs are
becoming widely used in treating cardiac patients. Cardiac "rehabilitation" is the new buzzword in cardiology. Patients who
have had heart attacks are being enrolled at an ever increasing
rate in exercise programs on the assumption that they will avoid
repeated heart attacks, or if they do have another attack, it will
be less severe. The very word "rehabilitation" implies repair of
the heart, and people who pay money for such promises at least
expect not to be killed straight off by their disease.

Such promises can't be kept. The physical condition of heart
and arteries at any stage of disease doesn't improve with exercise. Even the best-designed and best-controlled studies show
no reduction in frequency or severity of heart attacks, no slowing
of the disease process and no protection from sudden death.

A 1975 report from Sweden covered 315 heart attack patients
who were randomly assigned either to an exercise training program or to no program.[2] There was no evident influence of
exercise on either the death rate or the rate of recurrent heart
attacks.

A 1981 Canadian multicenter study included 733 men who
survived an initial heart attack.[3] After years of follow-up on
matching individuals randomly assigned to either a high-inten-

sity or a low-intensity exercise program, there was found to be no significant difference in either the rate of subsequent heart attacks or the death rate between the high-intensity and the low-intensity groups. In actual fact, whereas 9.5 percent of the high-intensity group had repeat heart attacks, only 7.3 percent of those less active did.

A five-year World Health Organization study of 375 survivors of a heart attack who were randomly assigned to a "comprehensive intervention group" or to a control group showed that total mortality was not significantly different for the intervention group than for the control group.[4] Coronary mortality was reduced in the intervention group largely because of fewer sudden deaths in the first six months after the heart attack. Since these patients received more protective cardiovascular medications than patients in the control group, the reduction in mortality speaks only for the benefits of a comprehensive treatment program, not for exercise alone. Incidentally, there were more nonfatal recurrent heart attacks in the intervention group than in the control group, and researchers couldn't find any difference in either group's capacity to do physical work.

An ambitious study, the National Exercise and Heart Disease Project, was planned in the United States a few years ago to make a definite assessment of the therapeutic effects of exercise by following a very large group of patients.[5] Although the size of the originally proposed patient sample was eventually scaled down, 651 patients who had survived an initial heart attack were randomly assigned to exercise or to no exercise, and followed over a three-year period. The results, simply put, showed no significant difference in the rate of recurrence or death.

These studies are admittedly imperfect. Their design, like that of other such studies, can be faulted and the number of subjects analyzed is rather small. About 27 percent of patients are excluded from exercise training programs after a heart attack for other medical reasons, such as heart failure, uncontrolled hypertension or arrhythmias. Patients drop out of treatment groups unpredictably, and probably some patients who are not in the exercise program exercise anyway. Despite their limitations, however, they are the best studies available, and the inescapable conclusion is that they show no secondary prevention at the early stages of disease, no tertiary prevention after symptoms are obvious—in fact, no benefits from exercise at all.

When the claims of primary, secondary and tertiary protection against coronary heart disease are dismissed, there is still a traditional and widely held view that exercise increases the coronary collateral circulation. Collateral blood vessels are supplementary channels that provide connections among the main arteries and their branches and result in an increase in blood flow. Coronary collaterals connect branches of each major coronary artery to other branches of the same artery, and they provide connections among branches of the different major coronary arteries. This supplementary system is of great importance in keeping up a flow of blood to the heart muscle when the major coronary arteries have become narrowed or totally closed off by fatty deposits. I have seen patients whose original major coronary arteries were completely obstructed by atherosclerosis, yet whose blood flow through their heart muscle was nearly normal due to their collateral circulation network. The fine interweaving collateral channels may be so extensive that the heart looks like it is covered with spider webs.

For years exercise advocates have suggested that exercise promotes the development of coronary collateral blood vessels. The major support for this idea has come from an experiment carried out by Dr. Richard W. Eckstein at Western Reserve University School of Medicine in 1957.[6] This experiment—on dogs, not humans—involved a highly artificial set of circumstances. Blood vessels were cut and tied to simulate the obstruction and reduced blood flow in atherosclerosis. Tubes, reservoirs of fluid and measuring devices were introduced into the altered arteries or connected to the circulatory system. The data indicated, according to Dr. Eckstein, that arterial narrowing results in collateral development proportional to the degree of narrowing—that much of his interpretation has been verified repeatedly by studies of animals and humans under less artificial conditions, and is now well accepted—and, second, that exercise leads to greater blood flow. This latter conclusion has not only *not* been confirmed, but an impressive amount of scientific evidence contradicts it.

In an important study of whether exercise would increase coronary collateral blood flow, Dr. Andre Nolewajka and his colleagues at the University of Western Ontario, Canada, studied 20 patients following a heart attack.[7] Randomly assigning 10 of the subjects to an exercise program and 10 to a control nonexercise group, and using highly sophisticated techniques to measure how much blood flowed through the heart muscle, they showed that both groups had similar extent and progression of coronary artery disease, and that neither group showed changes in the network of collateral blood vessels or the amount of blood flowing through the heart muscle. The researchers concluded that exercise does not affect the progression of coronary artery disease, the amount of blood flow to the heart muscle or the development of collateral blood vessels. Another study of the effects of exercise training, on 16 men with coronary artery disease, reported in the *American Journal of Cardiology,* showed that it failed to have a significant effect on heart muscle blood flow.[8] Angiographic studies (films of dye injections into the coronary arteries) by still other researchers have not shown any increase in coronary blood flow in either trained athletes or as a result of exercise in ordinary people or patients with heart disease.

The consensus of experts is that there is no evidence that exercise training increases the coronary collateral circulation in humans. When collateral circulation improves subsequent to training, it appears to be coincidence. The improvement is solely the body's response to increasingly narrowed coronary arteries as the disease progresses, and happens with or without the patient so much as lifting a finger. The only stimulus for new growth of collateral coronary arteries is severe coronary disease; the only way to grow new coronary channels is for your old ones to get worse.

If prevention doesn't work, and coronary circulation isn't improved, exercise advocates can still retreat to the highly publicized position that exercise can benefit your health indirectly by cutting down on factors that put you at risk for disease in the first place. Scientists, again resorting to technical nomenclature, categorize risk factors into "primary" and "secondary" ones. Primary risk factors are those with a clear-cut and independent statistical relationship to the development of coronary artery disease. In other words, the presence of any one of the primary risk factors leads to the occurrence of coronary heart disease more frequently than mere chance or coincidence could explain. Primary risk factors are high blood pressure (hypertension), high blood cholesterol level (hypercholesterolemia) and cigarette smoking.

Each of the primary risk factors has been shown unequivocally to be related to the development of coronary artery disease. Your chances of getting the disease are above the average if your blood pressure is over 140/90, if you have high levels of cholesterol or if you smoke cigarettes. The higher the blood pressure, the higher the cholesterol level and the more you smoke, the progressively greater are the risks. Not only does each risk factor independently contribute to your chances of getting coronary heart disease, but also they are synergistic. Their effects are more than just additive. The risk of developing coronary disease if you smoke a lot, for example, may be twice that of a nonsmoker; if you have hypertension, too, the risks may more than quadruple. And if your blood cholesterol level is also too high, your risk of getting coronary disease may be nine to fifteen times that of a person with none of these risk factors.

Secondary risk factors are those with a much less certain and less independent relationship to coronary disease. They include obesity, diabetes, stress, abnormal electrocardiograms, socioeconomic status and, most important for the purposes of our discussion, physical inactivity. Most physicians accept the voluminous data relating heart disease to primary risk factors, for nearly every study that has been done has shown the same statistical relationship between the development of coronary artery disease and the presence of one or more of these risk factors. The situation regarding the secondary risk factors is less certain, for their effects on cardiac health are far less clear. The secondary risk factors are therefore often "weighted"—ranked in order of apparent importance—by physicians and researchers. When this is done, physical inactivity almost always ranks among the least important.

Scientists have pointed out that physical inactivity does not necessarily precede the formation of fatty obstructions in the arteries, and many studies have not found physical inactivity to be a risk factor at all. For example, Dr. Ray H. Rosenman, a California cardiologist, studied 2,635 federal employees.[9] He couldn't find any risk from physical inactivity. When Dr. L. Wilhelmsen, of Sweden, analyzed several risk factors together, he found that inactive people often happen to be those who court danger by being overweight and/or smoking too much.[10] Staying put may be *associated* with heart disease, but it doesn't make it responsible. The smoking and eating people do as they sit may be more directly related to heart disease than the sitting itself.

The most encouraging view of the risk-factor thesis is that, because both primary and secondary risks are largely under our control, we should be able to avoid heart attacks by avoiding some of the risks that are statistically related to heart disease. In recent years some studies have shown that lowering blood pressure, reducing blood cholesterol levels and eliminating cigarette smoking all lead to fewer coronary attacks and less deadly ones. Dr. Jeremiah Stamler, of Northwestern University Medical School, suggests that we can thank the antismoking campaign for 50 percent of the decrease in cardiovascular mortality in the United States in the last 15 or 20 years, the move away from high-cholesterol foods and other ways of reducing cholesterol for 25 percent and better control of high blood pressure for another 25 percent.[11] Nevertheless, there is less agreement that a person can be assured of fewer and milder coronary attacks by controlling risk factors than there is consensus that the risk factors, when they are present, predispose a person to suffering coronary events.

When it comes to exercise as a means of reducing risk factors, there is less agreement still. For here the data are even less convincing. The thesis that exercise favorably alters the major coronary heart disease risk factors is far from proven. Studies have shown conflicting results, and the interpretation of the data varies among observers. Nonetheless, the thesis has many proponents, and it is sufficient reason for many to have jumped on the exercise bandwagon, if not to have joined the crusade.

Since the thesis is less strident and less dramatic than the belief that exercise directly prolongs life or enhances cardiovascular health, it is perhaps easier to subscribe to this risk-factor argument. The claims that exercise modifies heart disease risk factors are more modest than the claims that exercise directly prolongs life and prevents coronary attacks. And you can believe in the risk-factor exercise theory without the sense of fervor or suspension of reason that seems necessary in accepting and promoting more dramatic claims. The risk-factor thesis is a more tentative notion, claiming only beneficial alteration in certain biological variables that, indirectly, may lead to longer life and better health. As such, it is easier for exercise advocates to accept and defend. But its acceptance and defense can lead to the same mischief and dangers as belief in the direct, magical and life-enhancing properties of exercise.

High blood pressure is a major risk factor for coronary heart disease (as well as for strokes and kidney failure). Depending on the criteria selected to define elevated blood pressure—and there is still some disagreement among physicians on this point—it is estimated that 30 million to 60 million Americans have hypertension. Therefore, major public health efforts have been undertaken to find hypertensive people and to get them into treatment. The percentage of hypertensives under therapy has risen significantly, and therapeutic improvements in high blood pressure are among the major medical advances of recent years.

In spite of pragmatic advances, we don't know what usually causes hypertension. Epidemiological studies suggest that it is, for some people, related to high salt diets and to obesity, but when attempts to treat high blood pressure by diet alone are made, the percentage helped is discouragingly small. Since we don't even know the mechanisms by which hypertension develops, prescribing exercise as a way of halting or reversing the disease is no more than a wild guess. Studies seem to bear out the shot-in-the-dark nature of exercise as a treatment for hypertension. Although some studies show small reductions in blood pressure through dynamic exercise in treating hypertension, the improvement is minor at best. Moreover, experts note that the long-term effects of exercise in people with hypertension are unknown, and they advise caution. In a study of 50 competitive distance runners, "Distance Runners as Models of Optimal Health," there was a substantial incidence of elevated blood pressure.[12] Forty percent had resting blood pressure of at least 130/85, which led Dr. Harold Elrick, director of the Foundation for Optimal Health and Longevity, to suggest that daily, vigorous physical activity does not protect people from hypertension.

Perhaps the best perspective on the whole question of exercise as a means of reducing blood pressure is offered by Dr. Marvin Moser, Clinical Professor of Medicine at New York Medical College and Chairman of the Joint National Committee on Detection, Evaluation and Treatment of High Blood Pressure.[13] Dr. Moser says that controlled exercise can be recommended to improve fitness and to aid in weight reduction, and "possibly, to reduce blood pressure in a small percentage of patients." But, he says, "there are no convincing data that systematic exercise, even if performed vigorously 3 to 4 times a week, has resulted in significant continuous lowering of blood pressure."

The preponderance of medical evidence and sentiment thus seems to be that clinically significant reductions in blood pressure are not achieved through exercise even when performed vigorously and diligently. There may be a few individuals with mildly elevated blood pressure for whom successful blood pressure management can be achieved through an exercise program—controlling such mildly high pressure may not even be necessary according to recent evidence—but for the vast majority of the millions of hypertensive people in this country and around the world, exercise simply is inadequate and ineffective as a primary means of treatment. To the extent that elevated blood pressure is a primary risk factor for developing heart disease, exercise doesn't help.

Whereas the sheer numbers of hypertensive people and the relative ease of detecting them make elevated blood pressure of perhaps prime importance as a coronary risk factor, it is in the control of lipids (fats)—particularly cholesterol and triglycerides—that exercise is reported to have its greatest effect. The exact mechanism by which these fatty substances in the body lead to atherosclerosis is still uncertain. All we really know so far is that following some sort of injury to the inner lining of the artery walls, fats enter the wall of the artery, become incorporated into the cells of the artery wall and eventually lead to thickening of the wall and narrowing of the artery channel through which blood flows. When the arteries are so narrowed, coronary heart disease is the result.

Cholesterol and triglycerides do not travel freely as fats in the bloodstream, because they don't dissolve in the blood. Instead, they are attached to certain proteins; the combined molecules of fats and proteins are called "lipoproteins." There are many different lipoproteins, and they vary in their density or weight. There are low-density lipoproteins (called "LDL"), very-low-density lipoproteins (called "VLDL") and high-density lipoproteins (called "HDL"). The fat in the very-low-density lipoproteins is largely triglyceride, whereas the low-density lipoproteins and the high-density lipoproteins contain mostly cholesterol.

Much attention has been focused in recent years on the differences between the various lipoproteins as they affect the process of atherosclerosis. Research has suggested, but not proved, that the low-density lipoproteins and the very-low-density lipoproteins deliver cholesterol and triglyceride to and deposit them in the artery walls, while the high-density lipoproteins remove the fats from the artery walls. If this eventually proves to be so, low-density lipoproteins could be the major villains that contribute to atherosclerosis, while high-density lipoproteins might tend to diminish the build-up of obstructions. Some physicians, based on the work done so far, already view LDL and VLDL as "bad" lipoproteins and HDL as "good."

The clinical support for this belief rests on observations that people with more HDL tend to have less coronary heart disease, while those with more LDL and VLDL tend to have more coronary disease. It is imagined that HDL could be acting as a chemical scavenger, picking up cholesterol from the walls of the blood vessels and transporting it to sites in the body where it is destroyed and excreted. Whereas some scientists consider the absolute level of HDL-cholesterol to be of most importance in determining whether atherosclerosis will develop, other researchers believe that the ratio of HDL-cholesterol to LDL-cholesterol is, in fact, more significant.

Exercise is claimed by some to increase your level of HDL. If the thesis that high-density lipoproteins are good is valid, then anything that would raise the level of HDL should be of value. Unfortunately, the evidence that high-density lipoproteins protect against coronary or other vascular disease is not overwhelming, nor has it been definitely shown that exercise increases amounts of HDL.

When high-density lipoprotein–cholesterol levels are very low, the incidence of coronary disease seems to be high. When the HDL-cholesterol level is somewhat higher, the incidence of coronary disease is lower. But beyond a certain level—and not a high one at that—the protective effect of HDL seems to disappear, and the risk of coronary disease seems to be independent of the level of HDL-cholesterol. If you have very low HDL-cholesterol levels, then a little more seems to be better. But if you have even a modest amount, more just doesn't seem to help much.

Let us assume for the moment, however, that high-density

lipoproteins are good substances that help to clear cholesterol from the walls of our arteries and thereby contribute to a reduction in the risk of coronary artery disease. How strong is the evidence that exercise significantly increases HDL levels?

Of the few studies that have shown increases in HDL in association with exercise, those increases have generally been so modest that sober minds might doubt that they have biological significance. In many instances, the increases in HDL are even less than the errors in the methods of measurement. In some studies, levels of very-low-density and low-density lipoproteins fell as high-density ones rose, whereas in others the level of only one, or neither, of these lipid-containing molecules changed. In yet other studies, where, instead of measuring the lipoproteins, cholesterol and triglyceride levels themselves were measured, there were again no consistent results. And the amount of exercise necessary to cause changes in the various lipid levels also varied.

A number of studies show no rise in HDL levels despite well-controlled exercise programs. Two hundred twenty-three heart attack survivors in the National Exercise and Heart Disease Project were randomly assigned to an exercise or nonexercise group, and, after one year, there were no changes in either group in any of the lipids measured.[14] Researchers from Tulsa, Oklahoma, reported to the American College of Sports Medicine that a 12-week walk-jog program that did have a training effect on the cardiovascular system of middle-aged men did not change any of their lipids.[15] Moderately trained runners studied in Columbia, Missouri,[16] and highly trained young men studied in San Jose, California,[17] similarly showed no systematic or significant changes in fats or lipoproteins. Commenting on the surprisingly high total cholesterol levels and low HDL levels in highly conditioned runners he studied, Dr. Harold Elrick said vigorous physical activity "does not . . . guarantee low total cholesterol or high HDL-cholesterol values. . . ."[18] Finally, an important controlled study of 25 men and 23 women from the University of Pittsburgh School of Medicine showed that, despite an exercise program that increased fitness, HDL-cholesterol levels *decreased* in the exercisers.[19]

When measurements like these are so variable and inconsistent, one would certainly have to be a true believer to claim that any sense could be made of them. But looking at some of the measurements in the context of those who were measured, one can find a gleam of sense.

In a study of 81 healthy sedentary men randomly assigned to running or sedentary control groups, researchers noted that those who chose to run more, and actually did raise their HDL the most, started off with higher HDL levels.[20] Studies of HDL levels in exercisers may well be biased by self-selection: people who choose to exercise often have higher levels of HDL to start with.

Despite that gleam of sense, the whole subject of the relationship between exercise and lipoprotein levels remains obscure. Were better light to illuminate the relationship, there would still be the taxing question of whether elevating HDL levels is helpful anyway.

An editorial in the 1982 *New England Journal of Medicine* notes that no one has shown that raising HDL-cholesterol reduces the risk of atherosclerosis.[21] A report to the International Congress on Lipoproteins and Atherosclerosis in Switzerland showed a 67 percent decrease in coronary events as HDL levels *fell* in response to a new medication. And it is notable that patients with a rare disease in which they have no HDL at all don't show early signs of coronary heart disease. All in all, it seems clear that a high level of HDLs isn't necessarily a harbinger of good things to come, a low level doesn't automatically mean trouble and efforts to change the HDL level by exercise are by and large pointless.

In observing an initial group of 260 men for 25 years, Ancel

Keys, of the University of Minnesota, notes no difference in HDL levels among those who died of coronary heart disease and those who survived. Keys concludes that the current enthusiasm for HDL is "unwarranted," and that low HDL-cholesterol is not a significant risk factor for death from coronary disease.[22]

The third major coronary risk factor—cigarette smoking—has no direct relationship with exercise, but its indirect relationship is an important one. The incidence of smoking is less among runners and exercisers. Who can play a set of tennis while puffing away, or have the wind after two packs a day to jog four miles? More to the point, people who choose to exercise regularly are often characterized by their commitment to a whole lifestyle package that may well lead to better health. The same motivation that mistakenly drives them to push for ever faster speeds and greater endurance correctly leads them to avoid cigarettes and pay closer attention to nutrition. Even Dr. Bassler, whose original Marathon Hypothesis is largely responsible for the misguided notion of runners' immunity to atherosclerosis, today credits the lifestyle of the runner for the supposed benefits enjoyed by marathoners.

While doctors and scientists are glad to have statistical relationships between risk factors and coronary disease for guidance, they would be happier still to understand the exact mechanisms of atherosclerosis and the minute physiological events that precede the cutting off of blood supply to the heart muscle. Were the medical profession to have a complete picture of the disease process, perhaps down to the biochemical level, then intervention at even some very early stage might be possible. Indeed, that picture is beginning to be sketched out. Hemostasis, the biochemical system of checks and balances whereby the consistency of blood is controlled, has a lot to do with the minute details of how blood behaves within the coronary arteries, and faulty hemostasis has now been implicated in coronary disease. As usual, however, overenthusiastic exercisers have jumped in, claiming that exercise has a beneficial effect on hemostasis.

Under ordinary circumstances, blood is a fluid that flows easily through the veins and arteries. But should an injury occur—a cut, for example, or an internal injury—the same blood coagulates to stem the flow. Coagulated blood—a blood clot—is later dissolved. These necessary changes in blood are controlled by the enormously complicated biochemical system called hemostasis. Although not usually considered among the major coronary risk factors, alterations in the hemostatic system can have a central role in vascular disease in general and in coronary disease in particular.

Your hemostatic system is complicated. An injury to a blood vessel sets in motion chemical reactions that, like falling dominoes, take place in sequence until a clot forms. Once formed, clots do not persist forever. An active anticlotting system, always at work, dissolves clots once they have formed. There is a constant interplay going on within your body between the blood clotting and anticlotting systems. Various internal chemical and mechanical stimuli tend to activate your clotting system much of the time, and if not for your anticlotting chemistry, your blood would tend to coagulate in many areas of your body.

Evidence suggests that many people with vascular disease have an exaggerated tendency to form blood clots. Clotting of blood in the coronary arteries is a singularly important event in the majority of major heart attacks. A clot usually occurs in an already narrowed portion of the coronary artery, and is superimposed on a cholesterol-lipid plaque in the artery wall. Many such clots, composed of various cells from the bloodstream held in a framework of protein strands called "fibrin," are large enough to be easily visible, but this isn't always the case.

In some instances where heart attacks have occurred, yet no clot can be found, tiny clots called "micro-thrombi" are the likely culprits. Invisible to the naked eye, they also tend to have become dissolved by the time a researcher can check for their presence. Micro-thrombi are composed largely of platelets, cells traveling in the bloodstream that are responsible for plugging up injuries to blood vessel walls. Platelets not only act as physical plugs but also release chemicals that trigger the process of larger clot formation. Although you may be aware of such "response to injury" goings on only when you scrape your knee or stub your toe, platelets, blood vessel walls, clotting factors and the anticlotting systems all interact with one another in a dynamic and ongoing process within your body all the time.

It begins to look as though atherosclerosis represents just such a response to injury. The inner lining of arteries can be injured by many things, including chemical substances such as fat molecules traveling in the blood, body hormones like adrenaline and other natural chemical substances in the body. Outside chemicals like nicotine and carbon monoxide are also potentially injurious. (It's interesting, in this regard, that urban joggers may have blood levels of carbon monoxide equivalent to those of chronic smokers, but they get theirs from sucking traffic-polluted air into their panting lungs.)

The artery lining may also be injured by mechanical forces, such as the shear forces of the blood itself. Both rises and falls in shear force against the wall of the artery have been implicated. Sometimes the simple trauma of blood cells bumping against the inner lining of the blood vessel may produce injury. These traumatized cells may then release chemicals that further the damage.

Any injury to the inner lining of an artery causes platelets to stick to the site of the injury. There, the platelets release molecules that stimulate cells deeper in the artery wall to multiply and to migrate to the inner surface of the artery, causing it to thicken. Cholesterol and other lipids carried in the blood-stream are then deposited in this thickened, injured area. As this process—injury to the artery lining, sticking of platelets, thickening of the lining and depositing of fats—occurs repeatedly, the channel in the artery for blood flow is progressively narrowed. Finally, platelets not only stick to the injured inner surface of the artery, but they form clumps, which release still other chemicals that lead to the mass of coagulated blood called a clot. At this point, if not earlier, when platelets have formed only micro-thrombi, a heart attack is likely.

Some claim that exercise affects the hemostatic process by tilting the balance away from clotting and toward the dissolving of clots, a change that could be viewed as favorable, at least by potential victims of coronary artery disease. If the claim were firmly supported by scientific evidence, it could be a reasonable justification for jumping into sneakers and sweat pants. The evidence, however, is far from convincing and even suggests that exercise may sometimes tilt hemostasis the other way, to-ward clotting rather than anticlotting.

In one study, clumping together of platelets stimulated by adrenaline decreased in a small number of exercising men, but, in spite of the fact that only the exercise aspect of the program was well publicized, their regimen also included dietary modi-fication and abstinence from smoking, so benefits can't fairly be attributed to exercise alone.[23] The authors of the study them-selves commented that the biological significance of what they observed was unclear. In other studies, platelet clumping *increased* after exercise.[24]

And so it goes. The thirty-five or forty studies published in major journals on the effects of exercise alone on platelet clump-ing—one of the big steps in forming clots—have found variable results: some found an increase, some a decrease and others no effect at all.

The degree to which the platelets tend to clump may be

uncertain, but the absolute numbers of platelets do go up with exercise. Almost all studies of platelet number following strenuous exercise show increases in the platelet count, the actual number of platelets in the blood. Dr. H. S. S. Sarajas, of Helsinki, Finland, found that platelets increase to as much as twice their baseline number after both short-term (30-minute) running and long-term (marathon) running and prolonged brisk marches.[25] Platelet-clumping activity also increases. If the studies that show increased clumping after exercise are accurate, and there is an absolute rise in platelet numbers, and those larger numbers of clumping platelets also induce more active clotting, exercise begins to look downright dangerous from a hemostatic point of view.

However, it is the iffiness of all this work on hemostasis that stands out more clearly than any conclusions when all the studies are examined. Two more examples convincingly show that there simply isn't much to be said one way or the other about the effects of exercise on control of blood consistency. In a 1981 study on blood viscosity, or thickness, researchers at Cornell University and Columbia University found that sedentary people have very slightly thicker blood (about 4 percent) at rest than do trained runners.[26] Thicker blood doesn't flow so easily, and it is known that pooled blood—blood that isn't flowing at all—tends to clot. But after exercise runners had increases of 5 percent and nonrunners increases of 4 percent, leaving a mere 3 percent difference in blood thickness between runners and nonrunners as groups.

In a second example of baffling results, scientists at Duke University reported that physical conditioning enhanced the body's ability to dissolve blood clots under the artificial circumstance of having a tourniquet around the arm; they also found, but didn't emphasize, that under ordinary resting conditions the ability to dissolve clots apparently decreased.[27] If an exercise-produced increase in clot-dissolving ability is a benefit, then the decrease at rest after people have exercised must be a disadvantage. Since most of us—even exercisers—spend more time at rest than we do with a tourniquet around our arm, the results aren't encouraging for exercisers. With the interplay of clotting and anticlotting activity going on in us at all times, anything, exercise included, that diminishes our anticlotting forces seems to present a potential risk.

Exercisers have expected that their intuitive sense of gaining vigor from a good session of handball or 20 laps in the pool would actually show up through the measuring instruments and under the microscopes of science. There *should* be real physiological changes, not only in stamina and brawn, but also deep inside, at the very heart of the matter. This gift science has been unable to give them. The whole scientific community, cardiologists like myself especially, would like to promise that exercise removes the fatty obstructions from artery walls, reduces the pressure of blood against them, keeps the juices flowing. But we can't. There simply is no evidence to support those hopes. As far as prevention of atherosclerosis or protection from its consequences is concerned, exercise will get you nowhere.

There is still another promise, widely offered and so powerful that it compels some people to run when they want to walk, to push ahead when they long to rest, even to drive themselves beyond the common limits of pain and exhaustion. That promise is that physical exertion leads to psychological, emotional and spiritual benefits as well as physical ones.

Physical fitness can make you feel better. But does it sooth the nerves and cure depression? Does it lead to greater self-awareness? Is there a magical union of body, mind and soul? Can you run in a spiritually useful quest?

6

The Magic Runner

Exercise has been credited with a wide variety of psychological benefits, from plain old "feelin' good" to euphoria that verges on the mystical. Since these effects are inherently subjective they defy easy measurement. How do you measure the amount of "good" a person feels? And when you can—psychological testing does seem to measure something—you can't say for sure where the goodness has come from.

Nevertheless, the simple good feeling that comes with a little sweat is so well known to most of us as to be unarguable. I feel good after a set of tennis, and my beer tastes better after an afternoon walk on the beach. Maybe pulling weeds does that for you, or maybe it takes a two-mile run. Whatever kind or amount of effort it takes, working for a while a little closer to your physical capacity usually brings a certain pleasure.

But even this lowest level of emotional benefit isn't universal. There are those who abhor a drop of perspiration and don't feel the least comfort in being pushed to exercise. Their degree of pleasure doesn't parallel their bodies' oxygen consumption;

exercise for them is a "downer." They may get the same comfortable and pleasant feelings others get from exercise by reading a good book or craftily checkmating an opponent in the cool recesses of a chess club.

There's nothing wrong with the experience of those who hate to exercise, and there's nothing inherently right about the experience of those who love to. Simple experience, for each of us, simply is what it is. To assume that all people will get pleasure from what pleases you is as foolish as assuming your children will eat their spinach because you happen to love it. Your delight and their distaste are equally valid, and equally unarguable.

At the next level, however, exercisers claim therapeutic benefits, such as relief from anxiety and depression. Here the promises become questionable, and the need for objective standards becomes more evident. If a person in emotional distress is misled by baseless promises, that is a cruelty that should be stopped; if the benefits are real, exercise is a most appealing therapy.

The idea that physical exercise confers a variety of therapeutic benefits is neither new nor outlandish. A number of experiments and studies carried out over the past several years have reported exercise-associated improvements in intellectual, emotional and social areas, especially in people judged to be suffering psychological distress. And the subpopulations of chronically anxious or depressed people are a major mental-health problem. Most investigation has concentrated on the question of whether physical exercise might alleviate depression and anxiety. Psychological testing has established some measures of these subjective states. There are problems, though, in evaluating such studies and drawing conclusions that can be applied across the board to the population in general.

First, there is disagreement on what constitutes a psychologically healthy individual.

The day may come when we can biochemically assess the

huge variety of hormones and brain transmitter molecules that ultimately control our subjective feelings, analyze their interactions and come up with an objective measure of just how good or bad a person feels. That day is still beyond the horizon. Meanwhile, researchers and therapists must rely on what are called "subjective tests," which, by eliciting a person's reactions to neutral stimuli, such as bland pictures or meaningless shapes, or by analyzing a person's responses in hypothetical situations, allow the tester to gauge how cheerfully or gloomily, with what calmness or fear, a person views life. How well these tests match how the person perceives himself feeling and whether they accurately predict what a therapist will find during the deeper probing of treatment are uncertain.

Besides tests for anxiety and depression, there are also self-reporting techniques for gauging such related aspects as self-esteem and social outgoingness. The results of the two sorts of tests generally jibe well: a person who is judged depressed by subjective testing reports evidence of low self-esteem and clinical symptoms of depression, such as sleeplessness, poor appetite and fatigue.

In a way, this correspondence between various test results creates problems in evaluating the effect of any single type of treatment. If a person's depression lifts after treatment, did the therapy work directly on his depression, or did it work by improving self-esteem, by offering social support or by helping him to sleep better? The problem of interpretation is particularly difficult with exercise because it has proved impossible to isolate exertion itself from the many other components of a therapeutic exercise program.

Also, although standardized psychological and psychiatric criteria for anxiety and depression exist, it's hard to relate our own normal everyday concerns to pathological states. The same measurable amount of anxiety that paralyzes one individual might lead another to get out there and do something about it. One of us might be immobilized by the quantifiably same depression that another of us copes with well. Indeed, anxiety that we can identify as arising from a cause that others, too, find reasonable—losing a job or having a desperately ill child—may be the healthy response to emergency that moves us to handle the situation as best we can, just as depression after the death of someone we love may be the healthy withdrawal that allows us eventually to reorganize our psyches internally, and to recover. If "free-floating" anxiety for which we can find no external cause or depression beyond what reality seems to explain can be successfully treated by any therapy, we have no way of knowing whether the same treatment would work for normal fears and sadness. And perhaps, because these normal responses may be necessary ones, we shouldn't try to treat them. The complexity of psychological issues makes measurement, interpretation and evaluation a lot trickier than counting platelets. We should regard "objective" studies in these areas with some skepticism.

Almost all studies of exercise as therapy show some effect on depression. A California study of depression in junior-college students in a semester-long jogging course showed that, while both men and women improved their physical fitness as expected, only the women, evaluated by testing as more depressed at the outset, improved their psychological fitness.[1] Analyzing the data, the study authors concluded that those in the poorest physical and psychological condition at the start improved the most, both physically and psychologically. This unsurprising conclusion seems merely to restate the obvious: the lower you are, the more room there is to move up, and the more you improve, the better you feel about it.

The idea that exercise perhaps alleviates depression best in those most severely depressed to begin with has been suggested by other studies as well. In a group of 58 beginning-level runners who ran for a self-chosen number of hours over a ten-week period, the most significant improvement in "depression scores" was by the most severely depressed subjects.[2] Since the subjects themselves chose how much to run, important personality differences could well have confounded results attributed purely to exercise.

In another study of university students, both normal and depressed subjects showed less depression following a ten-week jogging program. Again, those who jogged the most showed the greatest improvement and also were the most depressed in the first place; they had themselves chosen the most vigorous exercise. Because the investigators did not conceal that the purpose of their study was to measure the effect of exercise on depression, the authors of the study themselves suggest that "the subjects' choices may reflect their compliance—or their desperation."[3]

The results of any study of psychological variables tend to be influenced by the psychological make-up of the subjects and their expectations of the outcome of the experiment. A subject's pleasure in physical exertion or expectation of benefits may enhance his ability to get better, just as his distaste for exercise or his skepticism about its benefits can obviate any therapeutic effect. Belief that a treatment will help makes it helpful, even if the treatment is a sugar pill or a nonsense incantation. This fact has been well known to science for centuries, and has been named the "placebo" effect from the Latin for "I will please."

The placebo effect is not imagination, but a biological phenomenon; although its mechanisms have not yet been elucidated, scientists have little doubt that measurable biochemical changes are brought about through the intangibles of hope, belief and the kind ministrations of others—with or without the added allure of a dummy pill. The effect is, in fact, so powerful that these days no trials of new medications are credible to doctors unless they incorporate "double-blind" methodology, in which neither subjects nor experimenters know who is getting the medication and who its dummy counterpart. Only in that way can researchers discern whether a new drug has an effect beyond the placebo effect.

Double-blind studies of the effects of exercise on depression aren't possible—there is no "fake" version of exercise, or any way for either experimenters or subjects to be blind to it. Therefore, every study done is tainted by the placebo effect, and so is the subjective experience of normal people who dose their ills with exercise.

If you're repeatedly told by friends, family, professionals and the media that exercise will uplift you and provide emotional "highs," belief may be sufficient to make it happen. It is quite possible that antidepressant effects following therapeutic exercise programs are largely due to the expressed and implied hopes of the experimenters, as well as to the expectations of their subjects. Indeed, in one study of exercise as psychotherapy for depression, the therapist weighted the scales blatantly by jogging with his patients.

Furthermore, if you're told that a course of action will have a certain result, and you invest time, energy and money in carrying it out, you are not easily disposed to admitting that you did not achieve the result. You may even feel foolish and have a nagging sense that you might be lacking in something if you don't feel what others do. Few are ready to admit, either publicly among their acquaintances or privately on some psychologist's self-report form, that perhaps they should have bought a book instead of sneakers.

When people are openly unenthusiastic about physical exertion and when their skepticism about its benefits is high, exercise doesn't work so well. In one analysis of an exercise study, for example, the dropout rate was very clearly affected by the patients' feelings toward the exercise sessions.[4] Those who did not have a strong belief in the benefits of exercise showed the highest dropout rate. The ones who dropped out soonest were not only the least enthusiastic about exercise in the first place, but also experienced fatigue and perceived little or no psychological benefit. As in other studies, those who were enthusiastic also complied the best with what experimenters wished of them, and they benefited the most.

The same holds true for exercise as it relates to anxiety, the other major psychological discomfort for which exercise has been credited with benefits. Expectations and perceptions mediate a person's response to any given effort. In one investigation, the placebo effect was incorporated, though in a different way from double-blind trials. A number of adult males were randomly assigned to one of three groups: a standard exercise protocol of endurance running; the same exercise after swallowing a placebo pill participants were told would reduce the fatigue and discomfort of exercise; the same exercise after performing an innocuous relaxation exercise with the same assurance that it would reduce fatigue and discomfort.[5] After vigorous exercise, there is usually a transient increase in anxiety. When this expected rise in anxiety was measured, the usual response was attenuated in the placebo-pill and placebo-relaxation groups by the expectation that they would feel better, although measured cardiovascular and hormonal responses to the standard exercise were the same for all groups.

A small but very well-controlled study by Dr. Dan Epstein divided subjects into those who were newly to participate in an exercise group, those who were to participate in a familiar but sedentary activity and those who were to take up a similarly quiet activity but one that was new to the participants.[6] The purpose of this rather elaborate design was to take into account the possible psychological effects of simply starting a new activity, be it exercise or something else. Although Dr. Epstein expected that subjects in the exercise group would show significant decreases in depression and anxiety, as well as increases in body- and self-satisfaction compared with the other groups, his hypothesis was wrong. Exercisers showed no significant decreases in depression or anxiety, or increases in body- or self-satisfaction compared with the other groups; indeed, all reacted similarly, showing no particular change in any of the psychological variables measured.

Whereas some studies have shown exercise-related reductions in anxiety, others have not. Dr. Ferris N. Pitts, of Washington University School of Medicine in St. Louis, has even suggested that exercise can *induce* anxiety, both in neurotic and already anxious subjects and in normal people.[7] Dr. Pitts showed that lactic acid, which accumulates in the body during exertion, and adrenaline and its related compounds, which increase during exercise, can induce anxiety symptoms in neurotically anxious individuals and in normal people under stress. Furthermore, since symptoms produced by anxiety and physical exertion are similar—a pounding heart and breathlessness, for example—Dr. Pitts suggested that exercise could intensify such reactions.

Anecdotal evidence suggests that for many people everyday forms of activity may at least temporarily relieve the jitters. Expectant fathers pace, apprehensive children may fairly burst into physical activity and almost no one feeling unusually nervous can just sit still. This may be because fear responses mediated through the hormones of the adrenal gland ready the body physiologically to meet external challenges by fighting or fleeing danger. It stands to reason that if we respond to the warning of "butterflies in the stomach" as our body is "supposed" to—by doing something—we will feel better. Certainly some of us do feel less anxious after splitting a pile of logs or plunging though the surf. But if these surges of exertion bring immediate short-term relief, does that mean a routine of exercise can have an effect on chronic anxiety over the long term?

Many studies of exercise and alterations in mood involve relatively few people observed for rather brief periods of time, methodologic problems that render conclusions hard to apply to the multitude that has taken up exercise as a way of life. In a study by the National Exercise and Heart Disease Project, these problems were eliminated by using a large sample and studying the subjects over a long period of time. The study was also valuable in that it addressed itself to psychosocial health in general, including depression, anxiety, hysteria, nervousness and sexual activity. The study group was 651 male survivors of a heart attack, and these subjects were evaluated before exercise and at 6 months, 1 year and 2 years after exercise began. The results, published in the *Archives of Internal Medicine* in 1982, were clear: "This study indicates that volunteers . . . in an exercise program for a two year period do not achieve greater psychosocial benefit than do control subjects."[8]

Since there are contradictory claims of psychological benefit from exercise, we need some perspective. We are probably wise to concede that some people who try exercise as a therapy for depression or anxiety are helped, although that is a far cry from the idea that exercise is psychologically uplifting for all. But the point is not so much whether exercise works, but, rather, that it has no special property to recommend it. The mixed results of studies, in fact, seem to indicate that exercise affects mood and psychological state by means that have nothing to do specifically with the physiological effects of exertion. The important and unanswered question is: Wouldn't anything else other than a program of jogging, aerobic dancing or other workouts accomplish as much?

When people have entered exercise studies, they have almost always entered a social situation. They may have been students who now run together, patients who now join together in a therapeutic enterprise. The mere social interaction—the banter and chatter among subjects, the concern for their well-being by the researchers, the exchange of opinions and progress—must lift the spirits. Isolation is the enemy of the depressed and the anxious. Give such people a group to belong to and fellows with whom to unburden worries, and some relief is bound to occur. Such relief also comes, however, by singing with a church choir, or by going fishing with "the boys," or by doing volunteer work in one's community. Exercise, if enjoyed within a group, has the advantages of some conviviality, but it has no monopoly on social rewards.

Social aspects were rated highly in a survey of factors influencing responses to supervised exercise programs. In an interesting study in *Public Health Reports*, Dr. Fred Heinzelmann and Richard W. Bagley examined such factors.[9] At the beginning of the programs, desire to feel better and healthier and concerns about reducing the chances of a heart attack were the primary motivations for people to join. The social aspects were rated as least important. In contrast, a survey of the participants at the end of the exercise programs indicated that the social aspects were among the best-liked features and an important reason for people choosing to stay in the programs.

A sense of mastery—the completion of a task, the accomplishment of a feat or the learning of a valued skill that once seemed difficult or impossible—may also explain some salutary effects of exercise. Such feelings of mastery are commonly reported as physical fitness leads to greater physical performance. Moreover, as exercisers become more fit they are likely to view themselves—albeit incorrectly, as we have seen—as less vulnerable to heart disease and death. Just as people who are depressed feel all sorts of aches and pains, those who believe themselves to be in the pink of health feel cheered. I wouldn't for the world put down strong backs and nimble feet as an avenue to feeling emotionally strong and flexible as well, but this way isn't everyone's way. Why not the mastery of a degree in social work, the nimble fingers of a knitter and the sturdy back of the trout fisherman? There are as many ways to feel at the peak of one's powers as there are people.

Exercise may also simply be a diversion, a time-out from worries and responsibility. How deeply can you worry about your work when you're worried about getting your next breath? Can you think quite as much about the kids when you're not sure you'll ever get over the next hill? Diversionary time-out from ordinary concerns, not exercise specifically, is credited with psychological benefits by researchers who have found simple quiet rest, vigorous exercise and meditation all equally effective in reducing anxiety. You'll hear the same from stamp collectors, potters and weekend carpenters.

While social interaction, mastery and simple diversion may explain many of the reported psychological benefits of physical activity, the very recent discovery of intriguing changes in body chemistry accompanying vigorous exertion has refocused attention on the physiology of exercise. Until late in the last decade, what little we knew about subjective emotional states, such as fear or aggressiveness, was thought to be mediated by hormones you or I read about some time ago in high-school textbooks—adrenaline, testosterone and so on. These hormones, which circulate freely in the blood, have very general effects and act on organs and tissues throughout the body. How they might be related to responses more subtle than the reddened face of anger or the palpitations of panic—to the pleasures of nostalgia, for example, or the stimulation of discussion—remained a mystery. Lacking an obvious bridge between the finer points of mental life and gross physical manifestations, it remained acceptable to distinguish between "mind" and "body." Mind was something that transcended physiology or biochemistry, and was therefore not subject to the quantitative methods of science, whose province was the body.

Beginning in the 1970s, researchers isolated a whole new group of substances, which they soon realized might mediate all sorts of activity among nerve cells in the brain, including those that control pleasure or the lack of it, clarity of thought or confusion, steadiness of mood or unnerving fluctuation. Mind and body thus began to come together—we are our biochemistry in spirit as well as in the flesh.

Among the first and most fascinating of these neurotransmitters to be discovered were the endorphins, opiatelike molecules produced within the brain that have effects similar to morphine on the central nervous system. Although little of the data accumulated so far have been confirmed, endorphins have been credited with shutting off awareness of pain in people who have been grievously wounded, have been linked to the pain relief of acupuncture and, some suspect, may explain the feeling of well-being that typifies some placebo effects. Needless to say, when it was discovered that blood levels of endorphins rise with exercise, there seemed at last to be a mechanism by which exertion could cause pleasure, if not euphoria.

The fact that endorphin levels in the blood rise with exercise, however, doesn't demonstrate that they are the cause of any change in emotional state. Dr. Peter Farrell, of the University of Wisconsin, emphasizes that emotional effects of exercise, if there are any, occur in the brain, but the human data on endorphins deal with levels in the bloodstream.[10] We just don't know whether the level of circulating neurotransmitters reflects the level within the brain. Also, to respond to neurotransmitters, brain cells must be equipped with the proper receptor, to which the transmitter molecule can attach. People vary considerably in both the quantities of endorphins they manufacture and the population of receptors that will accept them. And, finally, people's ability to produce more endorphins in response to the stress of exercise also varies.

Dr. William P. Morgan, of the Sports Psychology Laboratory at the University of Wisconsin, says that there is such tremendous variability in endorphin levels among different individuals both before and after they exercise that it is hard to see that neurotransmitter as the cause of a specific central nervous system effect.[11] As a 1980 review of the subject stated, little is known about the physiologic functions of endorphins and their clinical implications are not well understood.[12]

Perhaps most telling is a recent study reported from the University of Hawaii.[13] A group of marathoners underwent psychological testing before and after running for a minimum of one hour. They were given an injection of either a placebo or a drug known to block the effects of endorphins. There were no differences in the mood changes associated with running. The drug and the placebo acted similarly, indicating that although mood changes associated with running may be real, they are not mediated by endorphins.

Nevertheless, the discovery of endorphins has lent some credibility to the ultimate expression of exercise-induced alterations in psychological states—the euphoria that has become known as the "runner's high." We do know that morphine, so similar in structure to an endorphin that it fits into the same receptor, may produce euphoria in at least the early stages of addiction. And runners as well as some other dedicated exercisers often ascribe their perseverance to an addiction to the high they get when they push themselves to their very limit. One cannot dismiss out of hand what has captured the imagination of so many. Dr. Morgan and other thoughtful scientists are not convinced that a runner's high even exists, but objectivity pales before the magical vista of what *MD* magazine called "Unity with nature."[14]

Dr. George Sheehan has described the experience this way: "I had just attacked a long hill on the river road and had been reduced to a slow jog. Then it happened. The feeling of wholeness and peace and contentment came over me. I loved myself and the world and everything in it. I had no longer to will what I was doing. The road seemed to be running me. I was in a place and time I never wanted to leave."[15]

Dr. John Deaton, a physician, writer and runner from Austin, Texas, comments that one of the most desirable aspects of running is that it can transport you again and again to the "finest" and "truly pleasurable" moments in life, moments "memorable both for their intensity and for the fact that they are so infrequent." His running high is like the "first flush of euphoria that follows the taking of a central nervous system stimulant." Which, by the way, endorphins are not. At other times, Dr. Deaton makes running sound akin to falling in love. He becomes, as he puts it, "flighty with love and ideas. . . ."[16]

The lure of such poetic imagery can easily overwhelm a dispassionate view of what is possible for us mere mortals. Runners have surrounded their sport with what has been referred to as the "mystique that borders on the metaphysical."

A California running psychiatrist offers patients alterations in consciousness, euphoria and "changes in perceptions that ultimately enhance insights."[17] Kathy Switzer, the first official female entrant in the Boston Marathon, describes herself as "more sensuous . . . more physically sensitive to . . . everything." Not one to slight intellect, Switzer also claims that running makes her more mentally sensitive.[18] Dr. Sheehan describes sports and racing as "heroic," and refers to the "millions who are experiencing an escape to their higher selves."[19]

Eric Olsen, contributing editor to *The Runner*, writes that "the few seconds between the report of the starter's pistol and the final thrust across the finish line . . . are rich, and within them the sprinter will always find new worlds to explore. The perceptions sharpen and focus in on the moment at hand, the old division between consciousness and instinct begins to break down, and the flesh responds to the will with a clarity and precision most of us rarely know."[20] For whatever it's worth, runner Evelyn Ashford describes that same span of time not as a "sharpening," "focusing," "clarity" or "precision," but as a "sense of unrealness."[21]

Objectively speaking—which is hard in the face of such hyperbole—very few runners, dancers, jumpers, climbers or any kind of exercisers ever achieve euphoria. The sense of omnipotence and invincibility, of total relaxation and "Zenlike" peace, of either sharpened perception or dreamlike states that have been described will elude all but the very few.

We don't understand what a "runner's high" is, what physiological processes might bring it on or even whether exercise is the only way to achieve it. But one thing we do know: if exercise is a pathway to euphoria, the reward is bought at the expense of extremes of exertion.

The belief that the reward of a high surpasses the punishment required to attain it means that you must push yourself ever harder, beyond the boundaries of everyday risk and the limits of prudence. It demands that you suspend awareness of symptoms, of warning signals of fatigue and pain. The belief plummets you toward danger.

7
The Dangers of Exercise

Some of the dangers of exercise are only a little more bizarre than the hazards of everyday life. Runners in the 1980 Peachtree Road Race, held each July 4th in Atlanta, Georgia, reported a total of 61 dog bites, 3 collisions with bicycles and 9 with motor vehicles while running during a single year. Over 100 had been hit by thrown objects, including cans, bottles, ice, liquids and one bag of rocks.[1] Of course, people have been killed by falling masonry while standing perfectly still; you can't necessarily blame exercise for snapping dogs, flying rocks, freak accidents and crazy people.

On the other hand, over one-third of those runners suffered an injury brought on by running alone, and maybe *they* had to be a little crazy to take that chance. The kinds of injuries that occur to the muscular and skeletal systems in running and other popular forms of exercise are a veritable catalogue of orthopedic possibilities. In one extensive survey of records of 1,650 amateur runners with 1,819 injuries seen in just two years by two physicians at the University of British Columbia, in Vancouver, doctors D. B. Clement and J. E. Taunton identified 19 types of injuries to the knee, 22 to the foot, 13 to the lower leg, 5 to the upper leg, 8 to the hip and 4 to the lower back, as well as a number of additional painful injuries to each area that weren't diagnosed more specifically.[2]

Injuries in other sports and various kinds of exercise are also common. A random survey of squash players from two squash clubs, for example, found a 44.5 percent injury rate over their years of playing (which averaged two years in one club and eight in the other), meaning that just under half of all squash players are injured while playing.[3] About 10 percent were orthopedic, including back injuries, torn ligaments and tendons, sprains and inflammation; the remainder included lacerations and eye wounds. Contrary to popular belief, the better and more experienced players in this study had more serious and disabling injuries. Perhaps they play harder and take more risks—so much for amateur sports being "all in fun."

The problems of tennis players are well known—"tennis elbow," shoulder, knee and leg injuries. Most are caused by the abrupt stops, turns and twists our joints are ill-designed to withstand, not to mention the pulls and strains that occur when fancy maneuvers don't come off well. In an attempt to patch the damage and carry on, straps, braces and bandages are now probably commoner than white shirts and shorts on the tennis court.

Skiing injuries are so common they're part and parcel of the sport. A college campus after winter vacation often looks like an orthopedic clinic. And many an executive wears his plaster as a badge of honor. Orthopedic surgeons love snow as much as ski-resort operators do.

Dr. James Nicholas, orthopedic specialist in New York City, estimates that 17 million to 20 million sports injuries are reported each year, and that perhaps another 10 million go unreported.[4] Dr. Kenneth Cooper, who put "aerobics" up there with Mom and apple pie, estimates that 60 to 70 percent of all runners are hurt badly enough each year to cut back or stop their programs completely.[5] Surveys and studies of runners show injuries running—excuse the pun—from 60 to 90 percent.

Running injuries are especially common because of the punishing force your body has to take. The impact on each jogging step is two to three times your body weight. On average, your feet will strike the ground 800 to 1,000 times per mile. If you are a 150-pound runner, you generate and must endure at least 120 tons of force per mile. If you run two to four miles every day, you face from 720 to 1,920 tons of force each week. A marathoner may easily face more than 3,000 tons in a single race. Exposed to such stress, it's no wonder that muscular and skeletal injuries happen so often.

Knees are the most vulnerable part of a runner's body. The Peachtree Road Race survey determined that about 38 percent of new injuries involved the knees. Dr. David M. Brody, whose George Washington University runner's clinic has examined more than 4,000 patients, found that more than one-third of the injuries were to the knee.[6] Other large studies agree. The commonest injury, known as "runner's knee," is due to grinding of the kneecap against the bone beneath it. If you could see a knee in motion—muscles contracting, tendons and ligaments pulled taut, bones and cartilage sliding and grinding over one another—you would appreciate more easily all that can happen. It may be a miracle that damage doesn't happen more often.

The lower legs and feet are the next most vulnerable areas. Doctors Clement and Taunton found 28 percent and 17 percent of injuries involved, respectively, the lower leg and the foot, with various forms of inflammation and fracture heading the list. Dr. Brody also reported that lower leg and foot injuries are commonest after the knees. A variety of other anatomic sites—thighs and pelvis, for example—then follow as less common locations for running-induced injuries. The recuperative period from such injuries stretches to weeks and months. The disability, both acute and chronic, is often significant. Time lost from work and direct medical costs may be considerable. Even a sprain can sideline you for weeks; and a compound fracture is going to make you and your doctor long-time buddies. Of course, what conditioning was gained from exercise is generally quickly lost during recuperation.

Most of these injuries are avoidable. Runners hurt themselves by running too hard, or too long, or over terrain that is too steep, hard, rough or uneven for them. Other exercisers, too, get hurt by literally throwing themselves into the game. Damage to joints, muscles, tendons and bones generally results from overuse, not from acute trauma, such as, say, a nasty fall on an icy pavement. The practices that hurt exercisers are those they choose for themselves. One would like to think they do so because they are uninformed or misinformed.

Lots of people do injure themselves during strenuous exercise because they're unaware of just how easily injury can occur. They pick up heavy objects the wrong way, and strain their back muscles. They launch into a fast tennis game without warming up, and tear a stiff muscle unready for forceful stretching. They go out to jog for the very first time, and an ankle unprepared for the pounding of pavement "gives" as they turn a corner, or a tendon pulled for an hour without rest becomes inflamed and painful. Knowing this can help—if you're willing to make allowances for the limitations of bones, joints, muscles and tendons.

Whereas it's possible that some regular exercisers are truly uninformed, and don't see or hear or read anything about what they do, runners in particular are likely to have plenty of information. Yet sensible advice is overwhelmed by an overriding message: run harder, run longer—run for your life. Dedicated runners really adhere to the desperate idea that to protect themselves from disease and death, to attain the exalted sense of being fully alive, they must drive themselves beyond pain and exhaustion.

Dr. Sheehan boasts that he won't allow his body to stop even though he is "running on empty." When his hands are clawing the air, his legs leaden and pain is everywhere, he keeps running toward the finish he so "desperately" desires.[7] He finds the race the "moral equivalent of war," and he deems it "heroic" to demand of ourselves incredible effort "beyond depth of exertion."[8] A famous coach says, less poetically, "You have to run until it hurts." And another tells me that the real satisfaction comes from "pushing yourself to your limit—and then going beyond it!"

In the face of this sort of encouragement, some runners simply cannot run sensibly. The term "addiction" has been increasingly used to explain the dedication of a growing number of joggers to punishing activity. Dr. William P. Morgan, of the University of Wisconsin, claims these runners demonstrate the major characteristics of real addiction. They will do almost anything to get a running "fix," and they have withdrawal symptoms, such as depression, irritability and insomnia if they can't run. Although less studied, the same symptoms of addiction have been observed among other exercisers, too. An exercise addict will keep on going even when told to stop; he will ignore pain and take medicines or shots to relieve it. He may exercise, says Dr. Morgan, to the point where injuries are "near-crippling."[9]

Perhaps the term "exercise addict" can be applied to only

a small minority, but a frightening number of exercise enthusiasts act contrary to reason and common sense, as though im-
pelled by some demon of their own to disregard the signals
given by their bodies. In a survey at Toronto Western Hospital's
sports medicine clinic, which is available to all comers, nearly
one-half of the patients waited five days or longer to seek medical help after being injured.[10] The longest delays were found
among those who set the highest personal performance standards, and who regarded their activity as life-enhancing and health-
promoting. Clinic doctor Geoffrey J. Lloyd noted that the injured tended to minimize the painfulness of the injury and to
disregard serious symptoms. They didn't perceive obvious injury
as significant, didn't want to believe they were injured and were
reluctant to discontinue activity to allow injuries to heal. Even
James Fixx, author of *The Complete Book of Running* and the
last person to discourage it, admits that "when a runner comes
to see [a physician] with an injury, it's his last resort. He will
have tried everything else he can think of that might enable him
to keep running—including prayer."[11]

Of course, full-time athletes have become notorious for continuing in the face of injury. Doug Petersen, the Olympic skier,
continued to ski for three weeks with a fractured vertebra in
his neck; he finally had to undergo surgery. As reported by
Fraser Kent, a medical writer, he was quoted: "Deep inside, I
knew there was something wrong, that I was injured."[12] All too
often, such ordeals are viewed as heroism. Worse, these dangerous denials become in many recreational athletes' minds the
model they are to follow.

Dr. K. Wayne Marshall, of the University of Toronto, feels
that although recreational athletes may misinterpret the pains
they experience, they compound ignorance by "macho" stoicism. He has found that those who consistently endanger themselves by denying the significance of pain are also those who

"had set unrealistic goals. Their striving to achieve these goals often led to injury."[13]

An example is Jim Ryan, a television reporter and avid runner, who described his experience in a network TV news segment. He had felt pain in one thigh after a 10-mile run. His response was to run 11 miles the following day. After that, he could barely walk.

In 1979, television watchers were treated to the appalling view of President Jimmy Carter being forced from a 6.2-mile race by his physician, who saw him visibly faltering. And those who followed the Boston Marathon in 1982 may recall that the winner, Alberto Salazar, almost died of dehydration and low body temperature right after his great victory. Said Fred Lebow, President of the New York Road Runners Club, "If that kid had a choice of losing or dying, he would choose death."[14]

Physicians, who certainly cannot claim to be uninformed or unaware of the dangers, are themselves not immune to the suspension of common sense that leads to such a high incidence of exercise-induced injuries. A sedentary New York State physician describes how he ran the Boston Marathon: "I trained in two months, but I wouldn't recommend that. I lost 60 pounds and went from zero miles to 20-mile runs. I lost all my toenails. Blood was running out of my shoes."[15]

An overweight middle-aged cardiologist from West Virginia ran the same race with a stress fracture, coming in last—but proud.[16] And still another doctor, John Deaton, from Austin, Texas, decided to run an upcoming quarter-marathon even though he was just recovering from the flu. On the fifth day of his "all-out" training program, his temperature shot up to 105°. He self-diagnosed a relapse of the flu, but four days later wound up on the hospital critical list with lobar pneumonia. "The main danger," Deaton says, "is that the ecstasy you feel at what you have accomplished may lure you like a siren song to do too much too quickly, to ignore the soft whispers of caution that come from your body . . . euphoria and a feeling of indestructibility can override aches, pains, even common sense. The hurt comes later. . . ."[17]

If these are the exercise heroes, then surely exercise enthusiasts—beginner, novice and expert—are in for trouble. The machismo-tinted lenses through which we see such folly translates sitting out the last set of tennis or slowing to a walk when jogging as giving in and giving up. Nor is driving the body harder than it can take confined to would-be marathoners, or to men. Slow joggers who only want to jounce off a few pounds and suburban housewives who worry about sags and bulges have joined the injury statistics in droves. Women, in fact, are particularly prone to their own varieties of damage.

Special vulnerability to orthopedic injury in women exists mainly because of anatomical differences in their bones, joints and muscles.[18] Women have a slighter bone structure, with more delicate ligaments and tendons. The structure of their collagen, the matrix of connective and other supporting tissues, is different. Their center of gravity, the place where the body experiences the greatest force, is between their hipbones, making them vulnerable to pelvic injuries, whereas in men the center of gravity is usually higher, between the chest and waist. Dr. Dennis J. Sullivan, orthopedic surgeon at the Hospital for Special Surgery in New York City, found that five out of six stress fractures in the pelvis were in exercising women over thirty years of age, and there have been similar reports of frequent stress fractures in women from other researchers.

The wider pelvis of women—great for the exercise of childbirth but not for running—means their thigh bones stand at an angle and lean in toward the knees, causing unequal stresses on the inside and outside of the knee joints. Their knees are more mobile and their thigh muscles weaker, so their knees aren't held in place so well, making them vulnerable to knee injuries. Even among top-ranked tennis players, many more females than males suffer knee injuries.

Women's narrower shoulders and chests make them more prone to shoulder dislocations than men are. General body flexibility, although an advantage for dancing and gymnastics, adds to the risks of dislocation and fracture. And there is the additional element of inadequate preparation. The late Dr. John L. Marshall, famed orthopedic sports medicine specialist, suggested that the greater number of strains, sprains and dislocations in women who first start exercising are due, at least in part, to less prior training. And Dr. Howard A. Kiernan, orthopedic surgeon at Presbyterian Hospital in New York City, found an "epidemic" of knee ailments among jogging suburban housewives, which he attributed to "poor conditioning."[19]

There is also the disturbing possibility that something serious is going on within the bones of female exercisers. There is recent evidence, for example, that women runners may lose significant amounts of minerals, such as calcium, from their bones, and thereby develop early osteoporosis—a condition characterized by loss of bone minerals, leading to "softening" of the bones, pain and vulnerability to injury.

This premature loss of bone seems to be intimately tied to changes in female hormone function induced by exercise. It has been known for some years that there are interactions between physical activity and the menstrual cycle. But it is only since women in greater numbers have taken up physical exercise that hormone changes have been recognized as a general problem. Earlier surveys of women athletes suggested that about 10 percent had abnormal menstrual cycles. More recently, as women have become more involved in year-round training programs, the occurrence of menstrual irregularities has increased.

It's not clear just how exercise induces loss of menstrual regularity or even stops menstruation altogether. But it appears that when exercise-induced loss of weight reduces the fat in a woman's body to below a certain proportion, variably estimated to be between 17 and 22 percent of her total weight, menstruation is affected. Women who train the most and weigh the least tend to have few or no menstrual cycles.

Whatever the mechanism for exercise-induced menstrual abnormality, it seems clear that those women who stop menstruating do suffer from osteoporosis, just as women tend to do after menopause, when the hormone balance their bodies have been accustomed to since adolescence changes. Women with amenorrhea—loss of menstruation—due to exercise seem to be as much at risk for bone loss as much older women would normally be.

The consequences of bones lacking in minerals are fairly predictable. They're painful and they break more easily. Other, nonorthopedic, results of hormone changes induced by exercise are not well understood. Certainly fertility is diminished in women who lose their periods, although this is an imperfect means of birth control, because some athletic women without periods may still ovulate and become pregnant. (Incidentally, no unusual problems have been noted in pregnant runners. There is a wonderful tale that has circulated through medical and running circles of a pregnant runner who didn't feel well one day during a run, discovered she was in labor, and ran the remaining distance to the hospital, where she gave birth to a healthy baby.)

Men and women are equally liable to thermal problems— the excessive heating or cooling of internal body temperature. While thermal abnormalities don't put you up in plaster or sentence you to crutches, they're medically alarming. Any exerciser balances the heat generated by activity with the heat lost through evaporation of sweat and other mechanisms of body heat loss. A combination of high-intensity exercise, high air temperature and humidity and body dehydration can lead to overheating, called "hyperthermia." The clinical expression of hyperthermia can vary from relatively mild heat cramps characterized by muscle spasms, through serious heat exhaustion, to heatstroke, which is life-threatening. With heatstroke the person's temperature rises to above 105°, his brain is affected, so that he is confused, delirious or falls into a coma, followed by circulatory collapse and even death. Needless to say, unaccompanied exercisers are at great risk; once confused, they often can't seek help. When the temperature and humidity climb into the 90s, exercisers—and that means bikers and tennis players as well as joggers—should probably take a swim instead.

The opposite end of the thermal injury spectrum is "hypothermia," body temperature that is too low. Overcooling is just as serious as overheating. When the weather is cold, and lightly clad exercisers sweat heavily in a prolonged effort, their body temperature may drop markedly. If body temperature falls below about 90°, irrational behavior, loss of coordination and confusion may occur; the victim may, however, remain unaware of his own symptoms—again a reason to not exercise alone. In severe cases, respiratory insufficiency, cardiac rhythm irregularities and dangerously low blood pressure follow. Hypothermia, too, can end in death.

A few people are even allergic to exercise, or at least are felled by the same syndrome, called "anaphylaxis," which is the most serious allergic reaction in those who are sensitive to, say, shellfish or bee stings. Why some people should bring on this sudden loss of blood pressure, swelling of the throat and inability to breathe simply by exerting themselves is unknown. In a report of 16 patients suffering life-threatening anaphylaxis, the attacks were precipitated by jogging, running, playing soccer, basketball or tennis and even by dancing.[20] The syndrome can occur without any previous history or symptoms of allergy, in novice as well as trained athletes, and training does not decrease the likelihood of it occurring.

Another allergic-type reaction is called "exercise-induced asthma." Those with a history of asthma may already be aware that breathing in cold air or exerting themselves too much may bring on this spasm of the lower bronchial tubes. About 2 percent of the general population has such a history, but a lot of other people who have never had classic asthma are also susceptible to asthma provoked by exercise. Although any exertion may precipitate it, running is the commonest, probably due to the cooling of bronchial air passages during rapid breathing. Some researchers believe physical exertion itself, even without cooling of the bronchial tubes, may stimulate the secretion of a spasm-producing substance.

"Runner's anemia," or "sports anemia," deserves mention because so many people are aware of it, and concerned. It's a reduction in the number of red blood cells and hemoglobin (the protein within red blood cells that carries oxygen) of exercising athletes.

Since there doesn't seem to be anything wrong with the runner's ability to produce red blood cells or hemoglobin, the more likely explanation is that an excessive number of the blood cells are destroyed during running. The trauma to the blood cells by feet pounding on the ground is the likeliest explanation, a theory supported by the fascinating case of a man confined in a mental institution who became anemic by constantly pounding his forehead with his hands. Some researchers, on the other hand, believe the anemia is a physiologic adaptation, which, by diluting the blood, allows it to flow more easily. While runner's anemia is fairly common, it's generally mild, and performance doesn't seem to be hampered.

Exercisers often pursue their goals in spite of small nuisances like sniffles and coughs. Such garden-variety ailments, we are told, will go away in six days with treatment, and in half a dozen days without. Unfortunately, a whole host of viral infections, including the common cold and flu, can cause an inflammation of the heart muscle known as "myocarditis," an often serious, smoldering and permanently damaging disease.

The person with myocarditis, though sneezing and aching with the usual symptoms of mild respiratory infection, may be quite unaware that his heart has been affected. When viruses find their way to the heart muscle, they are usually few enough in number and don't make their presence known. We do not even know how many people may have had myocarditis with so little effect at the time and so little damage remaining that the disease has never been suspected.

When a person with myocarditis exercises, however, viruses in the heart muscle may multiply. As they increase in number, they cause more inflammation and damage to the heart muscle. The more acute the damage, the more likely is permanent scarring. And it is now believed that many cases of otherwise unexplained chronic heart failure—weakness of the heart muscle and inability to pump blood—are due to earlier episodes of viral myocarditis, perhaps unfelt at the time and many years in the past.

Those who "work off" minor viral ailments may be courting a chronic heart condition in their later years, and even an acute, sometimes fatal, exacerbation of myocarditis in the present. An example is a thirty-one-year-old man who was training for a marathon. A few weeks before the race, he felt tired, developed sniffles and mild muscle aches—the usual symptoms of various "bugs" we are all susceptible to. He continued to run daily even when, three days before the race, he began to experience nausea and a vague discomfort in his chest while running. By the day of the marathon he felt even worse and had to stop at 16 miles because of chest discomfort and vomiting. He had acute myocarditis.

Myocarditis is a happier diagnosis than some other heart conditions, for many recover completely. But to exercise during any viral infection is gambling on the possibility of chronic heart failure in later years and, during the acute phase of the disease, sudden death then and there—right on the racecourse.

Most injuries and abnormalities common to avid exercisers are certainly not "just what the doctor ordered," but even myocarditis is at least rarely fatal. The same is not necessarily true of heart attacks—and they are a real danger. Cardiac catastrophe, in fact, remains the overwhelmingly critical danger of exercise. This is so not only because the fatality rate is high, but because the risk of cardiac catastrophe is not so easy to avoid as the risk of tendonitis or heatstroke. People with coronary heart disease, even of severe degree, can often comfortably perform at levels of vigorous physical exertion that are not safe for them; the warning signals of impending danger are not always dissimilar to innocuous discomforts, and so are ignored; and sometimes there are no warnings to heed.

A meeting of cardiologists a few years ago heard that the first astronaut who ever walked in space showed frightening abnormalities on his electrocardiogram that was telemetered back to earth during his extravehicular space walk. Since he was superbly fit according to extensive preflight testing, the physicians at mission-control headquarters believed that the electrocardiogram was an aberration due to the strange conditions in outer space. The astronaut performed satisfactorily, felt well and passed postflight testing, too; the medical judgment seemed justified. Not long afterward, the astronaut died in a space-capsule fire, and an autopsy disclosed extensive coronary artery disease.[21]

Not only is superb physical performance possible in the presence of severe coronary heart disease, but also the person may himself not feel symptoms. I know patients of exceptional fitness who have severe coronary artery disease. Even people with imminently fatal heart disease can play sports, exercise and run. They may have no symptoms and may be capable of outstanding physical performance with hearts that will kill them.

More often, however, ignoring symptoms and signs that usually warn of a serious cardiac event contributes to the all-too-frequent occurrence of catastrophes associated with strenuous exertion. An exerciser feels short of breath, weak, unusually tired; he ascribes his symptoms to a large breakfast, a bad night's sleep, an "off day"—or even to "the wall," as runners call it, that he must break through to get to his effortless stride. If his chest hurts, his shoulder, his arm—those are just the pains of the game. Were the person sitting in an armchair his alarm might be immediate, but in the midst of the pound and sweat of exercise, he expects discomforts. More pernicious, of course, he has been led to believe that he should push on past these symptoms. And if he has also credulously subscribed to the protective effect of vigorous activity, he may dampen apprehension with strenuous stoicism.

All such ideas, and Dr. Bassler's Marathon Hypothesis in particular, raise false and impossible expectations. And they kill. Any idea that exercise protects from heart disease leads people to attempt what they simply cannot safely do. The Marathon Hypothesis goes further, for, in order to obtain "immunity," it asks believers to undergo the punishing regime of the 26-miler. Not only is that itself a terrible burden on a sick heart, but someone convinced of his or her immunity to coronary heart disease is just the person who would neglect and ignore the warning signs of impending cardiac catastrophe.

Of course, if the Marathon Hypothesis were true, then a

marathoner could safely ignore the symptoms and signs that, in a nonmarathoner, would suggest cardiac disease. Crazily, no one seems to recall the full story for which the marathon is named. In 490 B.C. the runner Pheidippides carried news of the Greek victory over the Persians from Marathon to Athens—a distance of about 26 miles. Upon delivering his message, he dropped dead. Evidence from today's marathoners indicates that dropping dead—and from a heart attack at that—is at least as common among these "heroes" as it is among the rest of us. Doctors Bruce F. Waller and William C. Roberts, of the National Institutes of Health, in Bethesda, Maryland, reported on five patients who died while running, two of whom were marathoners and none of whom had clinical evidence of cardiac disease before becoming runners.[22] All five, the marathoners included, died from consequences of severe coronary atherosclerosis. The findings suggest, say doctors Waller and Roberts with polite restraint, that "Bassler's thesis that marathon running provides 'immunity to atherosclerosis' is incorrect."

Others have corroborated that fact of life. Doctors Timothy D. Noakes and Lionel H. Opie, of South Africa, reported autopsy evidence of coronary atherosclerosis in four marathoners.[23] Dr. Renu Virmani, Chief of the Division of Cardiovascular Pathology Research in the Department of Cardiovascular Pathology of the Armed Forces Institute of Pathology, in Washington, D.C., reviewed the autopsy findings on 7 marathoners who had completed a total of 64 marathons.[24] Four died of coronary heart disease; their coronary arteries were found to be severely affected by atherosclerosis. Dr. Virmani then personally studied autopsies of 3 other marathoners; 2 of them had died of severe coronary atherosclerosis. Comparing all causes of death among marathoner autopsies she reviewed, Dr. Virmani found that severe coronary atherosclerosis is the most common cause of death in marathon runners.[25]

Findings are about the same for less demanding forms of running, too.

Dr. Virmani, continuing her studies of running deaths after her initial findings from marathoners' autopsies, reviewed published reports of deaths of 57 runners, 43 of whom were joggers. Coronary heart disease occurred in 77 percent of the subjects and was the most frequent cause of death. She personally studied the deaths of 24 other runners—21 were joggers, of whom 13 died while jogging and 6 soon after jogging. Twenty-three of the 24 individuals had severe coronary atherosclerosis.[26]

One of the most important studies bearing on runners' mortality is that of Dr. Paul D. Thompson and his colleagues at Stanford University Medical Center.[27] They investigated the circumstances of death and the medical and activity histories of 18 people who died during or immediately after jogging. Fourteen of the 18 individuals had exercised regularly for one or more years, 9 of the 18 for three or more years. Although 4 of the 18 died during competition, most died during their usual exercise routines.

Thirteen of these 18 exercise-related deaths were due to coronary heart disease. As the authors state, "neither superior athletic performance nor habitual physical exercise guarantees protection against an exercise death."

Most of the victims had seen a physician regularly; exercise stress tests were normal for three of four people who had the test within two years of their death; the fourth was considered equivocal. In regard to the value of thorough medical examinations in decreasing exercise-related deaths, "our results," says Dr. Thompson, "are not encouraging."

Dr. Jeffrey B. Handler and his colleagues at the Naval Regional Medical Center in San Diego reported the case of a 48-year-old man with no known coronary risk factors, and whose testing showed him to be extremely "fit," who nevertheless developed symptoms of coronary artery disease after eight years of running.[28] Angiograms showed 99 percent blockage of one of the major coronary arteries. "Documentation of his coronary artery disease," says Dr. Handler, "and its relationship to his [symptoms] are unimpeachable . . . this patient remains the best-described example of the failure of a vigorous running program to prevent the progression of coronary atherosclerosis."

Other forms of strenuous exercise are no better at protecting against heart disease. In a report of 21 athletes, only 1 of whom was a jogger, Dr. Lionel Opie found coronary heart disease as the cause of death in 18.[29] Other studies have no better news to add.

Regular exercise does not prevent the development and progression of typical and severe coronary atherosclerosis. In most instances of death related to exercise, in fact, coronary heart disease is the usual finding. Dr. Thompson, discouraged that not even thorough medical surveillance could single out those at risk, summed up the problem. "Exercise deaths do occur," he warned, "and there is no definite way to identify asymptomatic individuals at risk. Superior physical fitness does not guarantee protection against exercise deaths."

Even the very young may die during exercise, although, unlike their slightly older counterparts, whose deaths are usually related to underlying coronary heart disease, the cause is most often a cardiovascular abnormality they were born with. Dr. Barry J. Maron and his colleagues at the National Institutes of Health analyzed the hearts of 29 competitive athletes who had died between the ages of 13 and 30 years.[30] Twenty-four of the 29 died during exertion, and all died of one or another form of unsuspected heart disease. The commonest cause was hypertrophic cardiomyopathy, a generally inherited form of heart muscle disease characterized by unusual enlargement and disorganzation of heart muscle cells. There are many forms of cardiomyopathy unrelated to the coronary arteries, heart valves or anything else in the heart that might produce damage. Not only is the cause frequently unknown, but the disease is almost as frequently unsuspected.

Even when heart disease announces itself, denial of warning symptoms is a recurrent theme in many studies and reports of exercise fatalities. Even the simple advice to "get more exercise" offered offhandedly by many doctors may be enough to make people ignore the signals that should be heeded. In Dr. Thompson's study of jogging-related deaths, 6 of 13 subjects who died from coronary heart disease had warning symptoms that they ignored, and none of those whose symptoms arose for the first time during jogging reduced their level of exertion.[31]

Derek G. Steward, a former world-class athlete, described his own experience with denying the symptoms of coronary heart disease.[32] After a brilliant athletic career, he retired from competition but continued to exercise regularly. When he found his exercise tolerance lower and experienced chest pain while jogging, he interpreted these symptoms as signs of "unfitness." He was not psychologically prepared, he says, to accept the fact that he was a candidate for heart disease. Finally, after pain forced him to stop after 100 yards of jogging, it became impossible to deny his true condition.

Severe coronary artery disease developed and progressed in this training athlete although he was capable of considerable physical exertion for a long time while his coronary arteries were closing down. Dr. Bassler's claim that it is biologically impossible for atherosclerosis to progress in anyone capable of even walking the 42-kilometer marathon distance is clearly untrue. Steward's experience contradicts it, as have doctors Noakes and Opie, who have documented the progress of coronary artery disease during the life of a marathoner while he continued to run marathons.[33]

115

The evidence is unassailable. Coronary heart disease develops and progresses during exercise training and conditioning programs. Exercisers die of heart disease despite exercise.

But it's one thing to die *despite* something, and quite another to die *because* of it. If the worst thing that could be said about exercise is that it doesn't prevent coronary heart disease or death, then those who enjoy the sweat and the pain would have no reason not to "go for it"—assuming the benefits of fitness outweighed the risk of injury.

But people don't just die in spite of exercise. They die because of it. And whether death is within seconds, minutes or hours after the onset of the terminal event, that terminal event often begins during or just after exercise.

Cardiac deaths that occur hours or even days after the onset of symptoms are usually due to heart attacks, where heart muscle cells are injured and die due to inadequate oxygen supply through blocked coronary arteries. Deaths that occur within seconds or minutes, so-called instantaneous or sudden deaths, are usually due to those irregularities of heart rhythm called "arrhythmias" that are so severe that the heart cannot effectively pump blood around the body. Most people who die of arrhythmias, like those who die of heart attacks, have underlying disease of their coronary arteries.

Observations that incriminate exercise as a precipitating factor in cardiac events are old and established. Even the weatherman is likely to warn his middle-aged or elderly listeners not to shovel snow after a blizzard. But to do a statistically proper job of finger-pointing, researchers have to figure out the number of such events that would be associated with exercise just by chance. Chance alone predicts that if you sleep eight hours a day, sit or walk about for another 15 and exert yourself strenuously for only about an hour, cardiac events should occur in the same ratio: almost all of them during sleeping or being mildly active, only one twenty-fourth of them while exercising vigorously.

The data from studies shockingly show otherwise. Sudden death was studied in a group of soldiers, eighteen to thirty-nine years old, who were shown to have coronary disease.[34] Fifty-seven percent of the fatalities were associated with strenuous activity, and another 38 percent with moderate activity. Not even soldiers spend 95 percent of their time hustling about. In a similar study, 29 percent of fatal attacks were coincident with strenuous activity, although the subjects spent only 17 percent of their time exerting themselves to that degree.[35] They spent a full half of their time either inactive or asleep, yet only about a third of the fatal attacks occurred then. And in a third study, 78 percent of fatal attacks were related to activity, while only 22 percent occurred with inactivity or sleep.[36] In all, a disproportionate number of sudden deaths were associated with strenuous exertion.

Other data confirm the same association of sudden death with physical activity. In one community study, sudden cardiac death was associated with activity in 80 percent of patients, including strenuous activity in 20 percent.[37] In another, Dr. Meyer Friedman, who helped formulate and popularize the concept of the Type A personality, reported that more than half of 28 deaths occurring within seconds of the onset of any symptoms occurred during or immediately after severe or moderate physical activity, most notably running and jogging.[38] "The close temporal relationship observed between severe or moderate physical activity and more than one half of the instantaneous coronary death cases," said Dr. Friedman, "makes us question whether it is worth risking an instantaneous coronary death by indulging in an activity the possible benefit of which to the human coronary vasculature has yet to be proved." It was also disconcerting that many of those who died during or immediately following exertion had been well accustomed to the specific physical activity involved.

If exercise had no specific causative effect on cardiac events—if chance alone determined the coronary death rate during exercise—there should probably be at most only a few hundred such deaths per year. When you look at the numbers actually reported, there is a dramatic causal relationship between exercise and death, a relationship that cannot be dismissed.

There are data that give us a truer sense of the extent of the risks. A recent study from Rhode Island indicates that the annual coronary death rate—that would include both fatal arrhythmias and heart attacks—from jogging is about seven times the coronary death rate during more sedentary activities.[39] The prevalence of jogging was determined by a telephone survey and the actual incidence of death during jogging was estimated at 1 per year for every 7,620 joggers, or approximately 1 death per 396,000 man-hours of jogging. If you consider that 30 million people jog regularly in the United States, the yearly cost is over 3,900 lives.

Other estimates and calculations of the incidence of cardiac fatalities during exercise are even higher than those given in the Rhode Island study of joggers. Studies of exercise programs vary all the way from 1 death for every 7,000 man-hours of exercise to 1 death for every 55,000 man-hours of exercise. There is no doubt that the older the population, and the more severe the underlying heart disease, the higher is the likelihood of cardiac catastrophe.

One Canadian study calculated an incidence of 1 episode of ventricular fibrillation (a quickly fatal arrhythmia) per 2,500 gymnasium-hours for middle-aged businessmen.[40] If a group of men in that age category were known to have atherosclerosis or its risk factors, their risk of provoking an episode of dangerous arrhythmia while working out in a gym could be as high as 1 episode for every 500 hours of exertion.[41] In a report from Seattle, Washington, 25 exercise-related cardiac arrests occurred among 1,957 men with coronary disease in a cardiac rehabilitation program.[42] Since a total of 374,616 hours of supervised training was recorded, the incidence of cardiac arrest in this group was about 1 for every 80 men, and almost 1 episode for every 15,000 man-hours of exercise. Of great interest, the men who suffered cardiac arrest were capable of more physical exercise than those who did not.

When you look at cardiac events in general—nonfatal heart attacks and arrhythmias as well as fatal heart attacks and sudden death—you could justify a claim that exercise is a public health hazard. The Institute for Aerobics Research, in Dallas, Texas, used standard equations for calculating statistical probability to estimate the maximum number of cardiac "events" to be expected in the exercising population as a whole, based on the events that had occurred in a sample of 2,935 adults who put in a total of 374,798 hours of exercise over a 65-month period.[43] Depending on the age of the exercisers, the maximum risk estimates for men ranged from 0.3 to 2.7 cardiac deaths or nonfatal events for every 10,000 hours of exercise. The risk for women was figured to be nearly double that, or 0.6 to 6.0 events for every 10,000 hours of exercise. Based on their statistical equations and their mathematical calculations, assuming that each exerciser puts in only about 78 hours of exercise each year (30 minutes three times a week), we could expect that between 2 and 27 in every thousand men would suffer some sort of cardiac event per year, and so would between 5 and 50 in every thousand women. Even using the lowest figures, if 20 million men exercise regularly, we could expect 40,000 of them to bring upon themselves a heart attack or worse; and if 10 million women exercise regularly, 50,000 of them are also likely to undergo a cardiac event. The lowest figures, of course, relate to the youngest exercisers, those least likely to have advanced atherosclerosis.

Attempts to pin down the statistics in exercise-related cardiac deaths and other cardiac events seem to indicate that, if anything, available data underestimate the magnitude of the risk. A number of cardiovascular complications probably go unrecognized at the time, and therefore unreported. A person may first experience symptoms as he pours himself a beer after a long workout or strolls home from the gym, and may not relate it to the effort he so recently put forth. A person may not inform others of feelings of weakness or even pain while exercising, so that the first they know of his condition is some hours later when, apparently suddenly and without any link to exertion, he dies.

Moreover, bad news is less likely to be publicly reported than good news. In one attempt at a survey of cardiac events at community recreation centers, 50 percent of the facilities failed to respond.[44] Although we can't know whether their reports would be less favorable than those from centers that did respond, I doubt they would be better!

As for your individual chances of appearing among the sorry statistics of exercise-related deaths, that is impossible to say. Neither age, nor results of stress testing, nor duration of exercise training has any reliable predictive value. Many people who die through exertion have done the same activity many times before without trouble. Superior athletic performance offers no guarantee against dying through effort. Perhaps the gamble is greater if you have heart disease, but there is an enormous pool of unrecognized heart disease in the population. Exercise deaths occur, and we cannot identify the individuals at risk.

We can say with surety that if you choose to throw yourself into exercise with the vigor and abandon enthusiasts promote, some sort of problem is likely to confront you. It may be orthopedic, metabolic, hormonal or cardiac; it may be mild or severe, temporary or permanent, insignificant or serious. But strenuous exercise is really gambling, and you have to weigh the stakes carefully. Do you stand to gain enough to offset the hazards? Are the rewards really worth the risks? Most important, is there some other way—sane, sensible, safe—to reap the fun of exercise without harvesting a crop of ills? There is, and it is available to just about every one of us.

8

A Better Way

This is not an antiexercise book. It's simply the other side of the exercise story, the side few people have heard and some don't want to know. The facts don't obviate the pleasures of exercise, but they do say exercise is dangerous when it's done for the wrong reasons. The truth can protect you from the claims and aims of others, and, perhaps, from yourself. You can't exercise for your health; you can't run for your life. But you can exercise for fitness and for pleasure, and you can do it safely.

Almost any form of exertion can be kept at a safer level if you don't drive yourself to overdo it. With the exception of inherently bone-breaking contact sports such as football and boxing, where inflicting pain and damage on your opponent is necessary for winning, even accident-ridden activities such as skiing and running can be done with less risk of injury. Take a less demanding slope, for example, or try cross-country skiing instead of downhill. If you must cover a lot of ground to enjoy yourself, trot, don't run. Cushion the impact on your joints with

122

good sneakers and see if you can find a soft running surface such as a smooth dirt path instead of harsh or uneven pavement. There are published precautions for every sport that is beset by muscular and skeletal injuries; risk can be minimized if you're willing to educate yourself in prudence.

More worrisome than orthopedic risks are the dangers of cardiac events while performing all kinds of activities. To avoid these, the ultimate risks, there is only one precaution that makes sense: Don't do anything to the point where you feel exhausted, unduly winded or have pain or discomfort in or around your chest.

It's smartest to plan to limit your exertion from the outset. That means long-distance running is not in the cards for most of us. Jogging may be all right, but only if you drop to a walk the moment your body tells you to slow down. If basketball is your game, half-court holds most of the excitement and challenge of offense and defense without the exhaustion of running up and down the length of the full court. Plan a three-set rather than a five-set tennis match; it ought to be sufficiently exhilarating. And if you're tired, sit out the third set. Later, if you want to play again, how about doubles? Planning your exercise prudently before you start will help you avoid getting into a situation where you suspect you should stop but the pressures of sociability and competition make that sensible decision appear gauche at best, cowardly at worst.

There is a subtle but crucial distinction between planning your activity to avoid getting into a predicament, and exerting yourself until the onset of symptoms occurs. Warning signals do precede many disasters, but by the time your breathing is labored, your chest hurts or feels heavy or you're light-headed or faint, you may already have gone too far to prevent an exercise catastrophe. Usually there is still time to pull back to a safer level of exertion; sometimes there isn't.

Even having reached the point at which symptoms are felt, it's still sometimes difficult to stop. In the heat of activity, when your own enthusiasm or others' eggs you on, risk may seem remote. It's just too easy, running the roads of your neighborhood or engaging your friends in fast-paced volleying at the courts, to put danger out of your mind and ignore what you might, under other circumstances, feel quite alarmed about. Aches, pains and heavy breathing are expected; they're all too easy to dismiss in the pleasures and striving of the moment.

Ignoring such symptoms is courting catastrophe. Denial of warning symptoms is a recurring theme in the studies and reports of exercise injuries and deaths. Experienced athletes and novices alike are guilty of such imprudent denial, and they are equally likely to suffer from it.

Then, too, although real trouble is often preceded by warning symptoms that can be recognized, that's not always so. Injuries, heart attacks, even death may occur suddenly and without warning. The all-out exerciser has no defense. Such catastrophes are unpredictable; prior training and exercise experience offer no protection. To exercise vigorously, to push yourself to greater and greater limits because you have no symptoms, is to subject yourself to unpredictable and unheralded disaster. By planning a more modest level of exercise you help yourself remain on the side of safety.

Some assume that when they are enrolled in a planned, prescribed or supervised exercise program they can safely abrogate the responsibility for their own safety. They feel they needn't worry about overdoing it, since the level of exertion has been chosen for them by others, who must have a scientific basis for the choice. Others, however expert they may be, can't feel what is happening inside your body. They can't know how much, how far and how long you should exercise on any given day.

In any exercise activity, supervised or not, prescribed or self-chosen, your best guide to the safety of what you are doing is your own self-awareness. Aiming for a predetermined duration of exercise or a preselected target heart rate is foolish if your body tells you that you're overdoing it. The pleasure of working up a good sweat may be just as easily gained at a heart rate that is, say, 50 percent of your maximum as it is at 70 percent or some other arbitrarily chosen level. And fitness can be achieved with less intensity of exertion than the rigid time-and-effort schedules outlined in so many familiar books and articles on exercise. Professional athletes need to adhere to more rigidly prescribed and severe exercise programs. Their livelihoods depend on it, and they accept the risks of their occupations as might a coal miner or an airplane pilot. Recreational athletes needn't and shouldn't, because the gains are illusory and the risks all too real.

Sensible exercisers espouse this idea: Listen to your body. This takes a bit of practice; you have to think about how you feel. Your body will speak to you in both general and specific terms. You know more or less, if you simply think about it—and you should think about it—whether you have a general feeling of well-being or not. If you feel sick in a general way, if you have a sense that you aren't well, you ought at least not to exercise until that feeling goes or its cause is determined not to be related to your physical health. Just because you can't pinpoint a specific ache or pain or other symptom doesn't mean that everything is all right. If you feel you're just not right, or are unusually fatigued, indulge that feeling and stop what you're doing. General feelings about yourself are important and worth listening to. As you exercise, think periodically about how you feel. Appropriate exercise shouldn't make you feel sick in any way.

Specific symptoms are perhaps harder to interpret because

with exercise you expect to breathe harder, to feel your heart pump, to have your muscles ache somewhat. The best guideline as to what is normal and what may signal danger is your own experience of how your body has usually responded to exertion.

If you think you're breathing harder than seems appropriate for an accustomed activity, for example, and especially if you feel uncomfortable breathing, stop the exercise. Pains in areas not directly involved in exercise—an aching left arm in a right-handed tennis player—are also cause to stop. On the other hand, if you feel mild pain in the muscles you're actually using during that exercise, it's probably safe to ignore it. Certainly if your chest hurts and you haven't been hit dead center by a smash at the net, you should quit on the spot. In fact, any chest discomfort—pain, pressure, tightness or any unusual sensation—should be a signal to stop exercising.

Many committed exercisers take their pulse as a way of measuring their heart rate at intervals during a workout. If you take your pulse, it shouldn't be for the purpose of increasing your activity to achieve some arbitrary training level, but to keep yourself from pushing anywhere near your age-predicted maximum. Using the convenient formula for your predicted maximum heart rate of 220 minus your age, you can tell how close you are to that point at any time. As a general rule—even if your health is excellent—don't exercise recreationally above about 75 percent of your predicted maximum heart rate. If you have heart disease and you know at about what heart rate you often get symptoms, you should keep your activity at such a level that your heart rate stays well below it. Of course, medications may change this relationship of symptoms to heart rate, and this is a matter to discuss with your physician.

Besides the rate of your heart, checking your pulse is useful to detect any irregularities in the heart rhythm. Some people have irregular hearts normally. Exercise may have no effect or it may even abolish the irregularity. But some people develop irregularities only with exercise, or their basic irregularity at rest increases as they become more active. These can have serious implications and are other reasons to consult your physician.

Most exercisers are taught to take their pulse by feeling the large pulsating artery in the neck, the carotid artery. Although the carotid pulse is strong and easy to locate, pressing on that artery can cause a sudden reflex slowing of the heart and a fall in blood pressure that leads to a blackout. Occasionally exercisers press both sides of the neck at once in their concern to take their pulse. Pressing on both carotid arteries not only causes a more severe slowing of the heart, but also effectively cuts off the blood flow to the brain. It's really better to take your pulse at your wrist, feeling for the radial artery, and this isn't hard to learn to do.

Although listening to your body puts you in command of yourself, stopping when something alerts you that all is not well will not endear you to the exercise enthusiasts. They will urge you on, tell you that you can do more and exhort you to "go for it!" When you persist in slowing down or stopping, you'll earn, not their praise for your good judgment, but their disdain for your cautiousness.

This isn't easy to bear up under, but just remember that exercisers often urge on others because of ignorance. They don't know the difference between fitness and health; you do. They believe the promises of longevity and better cardiac and mental health; you know better. Spectators gratuitously urge you on for the vicarious thrill of somebody else achieving a difficult goal. Marathoners, for example, know the compelling force of spectators cheering and exhorting them. And those to whom exercise is business encourage you onward because it's money in their pocket. Why should you be their pay check? The strength to resist the urgings of others and desist from exercise should come from knowing that you're no longer a victim of myth, an innocent taken in by your own credulity or by others' claims on you.

The pressures to conform to organized exercise programs, especially those supported within a corporation, can be unusually intense. A corporation with a full-time fitness director reporting to the president is making a statement: it is committed to exercise, it expects you to be, too. When the company spends money for equipment and technical apparatus, when it pays a hefty salary to a specialist to organize "scientific" exercise regimens or contracts with outside facilities to do the same, your choosing not to join is saying, in effect, that you know better and that they're wasting their money and your time and effort. In a community where most people participate in an organized exercise program, those who choose to stand aloof may find themselves standing "out" in other areas as well.

Yet once you assume control of yourself, know your own body to be the best guide to your own level of activity and no longer allow others to set your pace and goals, you may find that the whole gung-ho atmosphere of organized exercise programs no longer appeals to you. You may begin to question the whole basis of such programs. What is there about a particular routine or special apparatus that's better than a less special, less rigid form of exercise? Why should you submit yourself to group pressure or to an "expert's" pseudoscientific monitoring of progress toward an arbitrary goal? Their planned and supervised activities aren't any better than your own sensible plans for exercise. And their goals for your supposed good health make far less sense than your own wish to be more fit, to lose weight or just to enjoy yourself.

There are two ways to combat corporate or community pressure to participate in structured exercise without losing esteem or appearing negative or apathetic. First, offer your knowledge. Fitness does produce physiological changes, but they are not ones that make the heart healthier, or that improve coronary circulation. Fitness is not related to health at all. Heart attacks aren't prevented by exercise; exercise may provoke heart attacks. And, if pleasure is the goal, there are other activities you prefer to group exercise.

Second, select and defend your own form and choice of activity. What is your goal? It may be merely to perform that amount of exercise that will prevent the small risk entailed in a sedentary life, or you may wish to retain a level of fitness you are now enjoying, or reach for improved fitness. You may want only to lose a few pounds. There's nothing wrong with any of these goals.

As for the form of activity, the ideal exercise should be a rhythmic and repetitive activity. It should use the large muscle groups of the body, especially of the hip and pelvic areas, in smooth and continuous motion. It should be simple to do and require no special training or equipment. It ought to be inherently easy to pace, one that can be done quickly or slowly, for longer or shorter distances and times, and at your own convenience. Ideally you should be able to do it almost anywhere, and alone or in company. It should be pleasant and it must be safe. And if it costs nothing, all the better.

Swimming almost meets these criteria. The only equipment you need is a bathing suit and a towel (skinny-dipping reduces even these minimal requirements). The action uses the large muscles of the shoulder girdle as well as those of the hips and legs. The motion is a smooth one, and there is little chance of injury from awkward moves, sudden stops or twisting turns. There is no pounding or wrenching pressure on any part of the body. And, although you can sink, you can't fall.

But swimming is a special skill, and many people aren't good enough at it to get any benefits. It often isn't convenient and it frequently costs money. Even if there is a pool near home or office, there is a discouraging inconvenience about packing up, getting there, changing, showering and then returning with a wet bathing suit. Swimming must be scheduled to fit in with other aspects of your life, and that isn't always easy.

Calisthenics and aerobic dancing have the advantage that they can be done at home and at any time convenient to you. Calisthenics, however, usually falls short of having a training effect. There will be some gains in strength and limberness but the usual start-and-stop motion of calisthenics is not continuous enough to improve aerobic fitness. Aerobic dancing calls for continuous rhythmic motion, and therefore can increase fitness.

Both these forms of exercise appeal to some because there are "exercise along" programs on television and tape cassettes that direct the movements and set the pace. That's another problem. The speed and vigor urged upon viewers or listeners can subject them to much the same risks that running would, although they are at least on safer ground in their own home. If you'd like to get the fitness benefits of aerobic dancing, use instruction for learning the motions, but dance to your own music—slower! Turn off the music before you feel tired; don't wait until some arbitrary length of time has passed.

Bicycling, too, is an excellent exercise and has the added practicality of getting you somewhere. Many choose to go to work by bicycle. Though bicycling is a continuous, rhythmic motion that uses the large leg muscles, it's hard on the knees. By the time many people are in their forties or fifties their knees are somewhat arthritic from normal wear over the years. The additional stress from bicycling can damage the joint further and can make what might have been occasional discomfort into a real medical problem. Bicycling is probably a better way mainly for young people.

The accident statistics for bikers out on the streets and roads are also discouraging. For that reason, some who enjoy the motion of pedaling and whose knees can take it use a stationary bicycle in the safety, privacy and year-round comfort of their home. Exercise bicycles offer you complete control of how much to exercise, because you are the one who decides how long, how fast and how hard to pedal. I suggest starting by setting the machine to no pedaling resistance at all, pedaling slowly at first and increasing the time from perhaps only a minute to about 15 or 20 minutes. Then the speed can be increased, giving you the satisfaction of watching more miles registered per session. When you're comfortable with 15 minutes or so of fairly rapid pedaling, you can gradually make the work harder by increasing the resistance.

The ideal exercise in virtually every respect is walking. Certainly nothing could be more convenient. Walking requires no special training once you've learned it as a baby. Any clothes will do. You can do it anywhere, even in the house, although the route may get boring and you'll wear a groove in the rug. You can enjoy the company of others, since you don't require your last breath just to keep going. Walking, like swimming, uses the correct large muscles for conditioning; and if you swing your arms freely and naturally, you get additional benefits that way. Your pace is obviously easily varied, and you can adjust it instantaneously.

The trouble with walking is it's so easy. It's so natural that it doesn't seem like exercise, and it's hard therefore to envision it as beneficial. Well, it does require a bit of specific direction to make walking really useful and worthwhile. Done regularly and at a good pace, conditioning can be achieved so that the body responds to reasonable physical demands with ease, without excessive heart rate or blood pressure responses and without unusual fatigue.

The amount of walking and the speed you need depend on what your goal is. You may wish only to eliminate the very small risk of a truly sedentary existence. Sedentary refers to a lifestyle virtually devoid of all but the minimal, unsustained physical activity needed to walk from one room to another in a house or office, or from house to car and garage to office. Even such profound inactivity confers but a small risk for coronary heart disease; physical inactivity is at the bottom of the list of secondary risk factors. Such data as there are generally suggest that the major risk differential for coronary disease is between virtual inactivity and only mild-to-moderate activity. Doing more than mild-to-moderate activity doesn't reduce the risks any further. Although the amount of physical activity necessary to undo whatever risk is created by inactivity is probably small, the actual amount hasn't been measured.

As an empiric judgment, I have for a long time recommended a daily minimum of one mile of continuous walking at a pace of three miles per hour, which translates into a mile in twenty minutes. If people can do that twice a day, I encourage it. But I believe that the once-daily schedule is more than sufficient to overcome the small risk of a sedentary existence. You can be safe from the risk of a sedentary life without being capable of running at all.

A three-mile-per-hour pace is not running, but it's not sauntering either. It doesn't allow for a lot of window shopping, but neither does it mean you have to work up a lather of sweat. It's comfortable, indeed often invigorating, for most people. Some, particularly those people who have been inactive for a time due to either illness or personal preference, find the twenty-minute mile a bit severe. I encourage them to aim first for the distance, then the speed. In other words, go for a mile at whatever rate of walking is comfortable; once you achieve the distance, then pick up the pace. More than a mile distance and a speed faster than three miles per hour are unnecessary.

If your goal is to become fit, how much walking must you do? That depends on what level of fitness you want to achieve. A twenty-minute mile twice a day can't train you for the superb speed and stamina of an athlete. But if you want to do all the routine activities of daily living comfortably, then you don't need more. You can increase your fitness over a wide range by increasing the distance and speed you walk, and by choosing to include hills and steps. A four-mile-per-hour pace, equivalent to a mile in fifteen minutes, is quite a brisk walk—faster than that is virtually jogging—and will certainly enhance fitness. The point is that by staying within the relatively safe confines of walking, you can achieve all the desirable goals short of high-level athletic fitness.

Remember, you can walk anywhere. The outdoors is great, but in inclement weather you can do it indoors. Some of my patients walk in the halls and lobbies of apartment buildings. In suburbia, enclosed shopping malls are an excellent place for winter walking, and indeed for summer walking as well, when the outside temperature and humidity are too high. Because the pace isn't so demanding, and others can do it comfortably with you, it can be most enjoyable. Company and conversation are easy, and the sights and sounds about you can be savored. And if you really have some place to go, you can "exercise" your way to where you want to be—and no shower or change of clothes when you arrive.

Walking is the perfect exercise for those who have heart disease. Many cardiac patients, particularly after a heart attack, are frightened of any activity; they limit themselves unduly, narrow their horizons, sometimes make drastic changes in their lives that leave them feeling useless, invalided and depressed. "Cardiac rehabilitation" programs have become popular as a means of undoing these usually self-imposed restrictions, but while some individuals enjoy the camaraderie of group sessions, many people don't want to be lumped together with other patients and may resent regimentation. There may be no program at a convenient distance anyway.

Walking will serve the same purpose. It is just about the safest activity you could think of. Anyone who has difficulty during the early stages of a walking program is probably destined to have trouble even if he or she does nothing. Almost all cardiac patients who are frightened of exerting themselves can actually do more than they do. When I start them on a walking program, I set the initial limits so low—perhaps one block at whatever pace they want—that they are easily achieved. Just accomplishing this little bit of activity is often uplifting for such patients. I then ask them gradually to increase the distance and then the pace, always more gradually than I think they probably can do. I stress that there is no rush to achieve any preset goals—there is lots of time, and the emphasis is on long-term achievement. As patients increase their activity without disabling symptoms the change in them is often remarkable. Their confidence soars, they regain interest in work and sexual activity, they think about traveling—and usually they return to all these activities.

There is no mystery to exercise. You don't have to be initiated into membership, to believe in esoteric claims, to practice arcane rituals. Whatever benefits the human body derives from exertion are yours whenever you take a good brisk walk or enjoy yourself—without pushing yourself—at some other sport you enjoy.

And if you can espouse the sane view of exertion as fully as others espouse the exercise myth, you'll be doing a world of good for others as well as for yourself. If you can make inroads on the illusory benefits of vigorous exercise with those who have been seduced or coerced into wasting their money and effort and lavishing their hopes on it, you will be helping to check a dangerous and foolish fad. If you can convince a friend that he has no better chance of living to a ripe old age than you by sprinting past you each morning, or a spouse that his or her strenuous exercise regimen is more likely to be a danger than a benefit to the heart, you could even be saving lives. Indeed, the exercise myth may be the first public health menace that can be combated without the expenditure of any money at all. The facts are in; information is available. The exercise fad is a folly and a danger. It only takes you to spread the word.

Notes

Chapter 1. The Exercise Marketplace

1. Fixx, James. *The Complete Book of Running.* New York: Random House, 1977.
2. Restak, R. M. "Erroneous Exercising." *New York Times Magazine* (7 Jan. 1979): 12–13, 26.
3. Greene, D. *New York Running News* 23, no. 4 (Sept./Oct. 1980): 12–15.
4. Morris, J. N.; Heady, J. A.; Raffle, P. A.; Roberts, C. G.; Parks, J. W. "Coronary Heart Disease and Physical Activity of Work." *Lancet* 2 (1953): 1053–1057, 1111–1120.

Chapter 2. The Heart of the Matter

1. Sheehan, G. A. "Take the Muscles and Run." *Physician and Sportsmedicine* 9, no. 5 (May 1981): 35.
2. Moldover, J. R. "Fitness and Health." Paper presented at meeting of the Medical Society of the State of New York, 17 Sept. 1979.

Chapter 3. What Stress Tests Don't Tell

1. The Committee on Exercise, American Heart Association. *Exercise Testing and Training of Apparently Healthy Individuals: A Handbook for Physicians.* 1972. The Committee on Exercise, American Heart Association. *Exercise Testing and Training of Individuals with Heart Disease or at High Risk for Its Development: A Handbook for Physicians.* 1975.
2. Epstein, S. E. "Utility of the Exercise ECG in the Diagnosis of Coronary Artery Disease: The Dialogue Updated." Paper presented at symposium, New Techniques and Concepts in Cardiology, Washington, D.C., 2 Nov. 1978.
3. Froelicher, V. F.; Thompson, A. J.; Longo, M. R., Jr.; Triebwasser, J. H.; Lancaster, M. C. "Value of Exercise Testing for Screening Asymptomatic Men for Latent Coronary Artery Disease." *Progress in Cardiovascular Diseases* 18 (1976): 265–276.
4. Faris, J. V.; McHenry, P. L.; Jordan, J. W.; Morris, S. N. "Prevalence and Reproducibility of Exercise-induced Ventricular Arrhythmias During Maximal Exercise Testing in Normal Men." *American Journal of Cardiology* 37 (1976): 617–622.
5. Sheps, D. S.; Ernst, J. C.; Briese, F. R.; Lopez, L. V.; Conde, C. A.; Castellanos, A.; Myerburg, R. "Decreased Frequency of Exercise-induced

Ventricular Ectopic Activity in the Second of Two Consecutive Treadmill Tests." *Circulation* 55 (1977): 892–895.
6. Graboys, T. B.; Podrid, P. J.; Lown, B. "The Reproducibility of Profound ST Segment Depression to Maximal Exercise Treadmill Testing." *American Journal of Cardiology* 39 (1977): 288.
7. Froelicher, V. F. "Exercise Testing-Screening: Positive Tests in Asymptomatic Patients. Estimation of Severity of Coronary Disease." Paper presented at meeting, Clinical Perspectives in Valvular and Ischemic Heart Disease, New York, Nov. 1977.
8. See note 1.
9. Rochmis, P.; Blackburn, H. "Exercise Tests: A Survey of Procedures, Safety, and Litigation Experience in Approximately 170,000 Tests." *Journal of the American Medical Association* 217 (1971): 1061–1066.
10. Scherer, D.; Kaltenbach, M. "Frequency of Life-threatening Complications Associated with Stress Testing." *Deutsche Medizinische Wochenschrift* 104 (1979): 1161–1165.
11. Stuart, R. J.; Ellestad, M. H. "National Survey of Exercise Stress Testing Facilities." *Chest* 77 (1980): 94–97.
12. Ellestad, M. *Stress Testing.* Philadelphia: F. A. Davis, 1980.

Chapter 4. The Case Against Longevity
1. *Statistical Bulletin of the Metropolitan Life Insurance Company.* Jan. 1975.
2. Segerberg, Osborn, Jr. *Living to Be 100.* New York: Charles Scribner's Sons, 1982.
3. Taylor, H. L.; Klepetar, E.; Keys, A.; Parlin, W.; Blackburn, H.; Puchner, T. "Death Rates among Physically Active and Sedentary Employees of the Railroad Industry." *American Journal of Public Health* 52 (1962): 1697–1707.
4. Shapiro, S.; Weinblatt, E.; Frank, C. W.; Sager, R. "Incidence of Coronary Heart Disease in a Population Insured for Medical Care (HIP)." *American Journal of Public Health* 59, supplement II, no. 6 (June 1969): 1–101.
5. Paffenberger, R. S., Jr.; Hale, W. E. "Work Activity and Coronary Heart Mortality." *New England Journal of Medicine* 292 (1975): 545–550.
6. Paffenberger, R. S., Jr.; Wing, A. L.; Hyde, R. T. "Physical Activity as an Index of Heart Attack Risk in College Alumni." *American Journal of Epidemiology* 108 (1978): 161–175.
7. Bassler, T. J. Letter. *Lancet* 2 (1972): 711–712.
8. Morris, J. N.; Heady, J. N.; Raffle, P. A. "Physique of London Busmen." *Lancet* 2 (1956): 566–570.
9. Oliver, R. M. "Physique and Serum Lipids of Young London Busmen." *British Journal of Industrial Medicine* 24 (1967): 181–186.
10. Taylor, H. L.; Menotti, A.; Puddu, V.; Monti, M.; Keys, A. "Five Years of Followup of Railroad Men in Italy." *Circulation* 41–42, supplement I (1970): 113–122.
11. Keys, A., ed. "Summary: Coronary Heart Disease in Seven Countries." *Circulation* 41–42, supplement I (1970): 186–195.
12. Menotti, A.; Puddu, V. "Death Rates among the Italian Railroad Em-

ployees, with Special Reference to Coronary Heart Disease and Physical Activity at Work." *Environmental Research* 11 (1976): 331–342.
13. Chapman, J. M.; Goerke, L. S.; Dixon, W.; Loveland, D. P.; Phillips, E. "The Clinical Status of a Population Group in Los Angeles under Observation for Two to Three Years." *American Journal of Public Health* 47, supplement (1957): 33–42.
14. Malhotra, S. L. "Epidemiology of Ischaemic Heart Disease in India with Special Reference to Causation." *British Heart Journal* 29 (1967): 895–905.
15. Punsar, S.; Karvonen, M. J. "Physical Activity and Coronary Heart Disease in Populations from East and West Finland." *Advances in Cardiology* 18 (1976): 196–207.
16. Morris, J. N.; Crawford, M. D. "Coronary Heart Disease and Physical Activity of Work." *British Medical Journal* 2 (1958): 1485–1496.

Chapter 5. The Inside Evidence
1. Osborn, Gladstone, R. *The Incubation Period of Coronary Thrombosis.* London: Butterworth, 1963.
2. Wilhelmsen, L.; Sanne, H.; Elmfeldt, D.; Grimby, G.; Tibblin,G.; Wedel, H. "A Controlled Trial of Physical Training After Myocardial Infarction." *Preventive Medicine* 4 (1975): 491–508.
3. Rechnitzer, P. A. "The Effect of Exercise Prescription on the Recurrence Rate of Myocardial Infarction in Men." *American Journal of Cardiology* 47 (1981): 419.
4. Kallio, V.; Hamalainen, H.; Hakkila, J.; Luurila, O. J. "Reduction in Sudden Deaths by a Multifactorial Intervention Programme After Acute Myocardial Infarction." *Lancet* 2 (1979): 1091–1094.
5. "The National Exercise and Heart Disease Project. Effects of a Prescribed Supervised Exercise Program on Mortality and Cardiovascular Morbidity in Patients After a Myocardial Infarction." *American Journal of Cardiology* 48 (1981): 39–46.
6. Eckstein, R. W. "Effect of Exercise and Coronary Artery Narrowing on Coronary Collateral Circulation." *Circulation Research* 5 (1957): 230–235.
7. Nolewajka, A. J.; Kostuk, W. J.; Rechnitzer, P. A.; Cunningham, D. A. "Exercise and Human Collateralization: An Angiographic and Scintigraphic Assessment." *Circulation* 60 (1979): 114–121.
8. Verani, M. S.; Hartung, G. H.; Hoepfel–Harris, J.; Welton, D. E.; Pratt, C. M.; Miller, R. R. "Effects of Exercise Training on Left Ventricular Performance and Myocardial Perfusion in Patients with Coronary Artery Disease." *American Journal of Cardiology* 47 (1981): 797–803.
9. Rosenman, R. H.; Bawol, R. D.; Oscherwitz, M. "A 4-Year Prospective Study of the Relationship of Different Habitual Vocational Physical Activity to Risk and Incidence of Ischemic Heart Disease in Volunteer Male Federal Employees." *Annals of the New York Academy of Sciences* 301 (1977): 627–641.
10. Wilhelmsen, L.; Tibblin, G.; Aurell, M.; Bjure, J.; Ekström–Jodal, B.; Grimby, G. "Physical Activity, Physical Fitness and Risk of Myocardial Infarction." *Advances in Cardiology* 18 (1976): 217–230.

11. Stamler, J. "Recent Trends of Major Coronary Risk Factors and Coronary Heart Disease Mortality in the United States and Other Industrialized Countries." *Proceedings of the Conference on the Decline in Coronary Heart Disease Mortality.* National Heart, Lung, and Blood Institute, National Institutes of Health, Bethesda, Maryland, 24–25 Oct. 1978.
12. Elrick, H. "Distance Runners as Models of Optimal Health." *Physician and Sportsmedicine* 9, no. 1 (Jan. 1981): 64–68.
13. Moser, M. "Nonpharmacologic Therapy for Hypertension: Is It Effective?" *Primary Cardiology* 6, no. 4 (April 1980): 11.
14. LaRosa, J. C.; Cleary, P.; Muesing, R. A.; Gorman, P.; Hellerstein, H. K.; Naughton, J. "Effect of Long-term Moderate Physical Exercise on Plasma Lipoproteins." National Exercise and Heart Disease Project. *Archives of Internal Medicine* 142 (1982): 2269–2274.
15. Freyman, J. F.; McNeil, D. J.; Alanpovic, P.; McConathy, W. J. "Effects of 12 Weeks of Exercise Training on Plasma Lipids and Apolipoproteins in Middle-aged Men." *Medicine and Science in Sports and Exercise* 14 (1982): 103
16. Londeree, B. R.; LaFontaine, T. P.; Goldstein, D. E. "Effects of Increases in Training upon Blood Lipids and Glucose Related Variables." *Medicine and Science in Sports and Exercise* 14 (1982): 104.
17. Oehlsen, G.; Gaesser, G. A. "Time Course of Changes in $V_{02\ max}$, Percent Fat and Blood Lipids during a Seven-week, High-intensity Exercise Program." *Medicine and Science in Sports and Exercise* 14 (1982): 110.
18. See note 12.
19. Allison, T. G.; Iammarino, R. M.; Metz, K. F.; Skrinar, G. S.; Kuller, L. H.; Robertson, R. J. "Failure of Exercise to Increase High Density Lipoprotein Cholesterol." *Journal of Cardiac Rehabilitation* 1, no. 4 (Sept. 1981): 257–265.
20. Williams, P. T.; Wood, P. D.; Haskell, W. L.; Vranizan, K. "The Effects of Running Mileage and Duration on Plasma Lipoprotein Levels." *Journal of the American Medical Association* 247 (1982): 2674–2679.
21. Lees, R. S.; Lees, A. M. "High-density Lipoproteins and the Risk of Atherosclerosis." *New England Journal of Medicine* 306 (1982): 1546–1548.
22. Keys, A. "Alpha Lipoprotein (HDL) Cholesterol in the Serum and the Risk of Coronary Heart Disease and Death." *Lancet* 2 (1980): 603–606.
23. Williams, R. S.; Eden, S.; Andersen, J. "Reduced Epinephrine-induced Platelet Aggregation Following Cardiac Rehabilitation." *Journal of Cardiac Rehabilitation* 1, no. 2 (May 1981): 127–134.
24. Green, L. H.; Seroppian, E.; Handin, R. I. "Platelet Activation During Exercise-induced Myocardial Ischemia." *New England Journal of Medicine* 302 (1980): 193–197.
    Kumpuris, A. G.; Luchi, R. J.; Waddell, C. C.; Miller, R. R. "Production of Circulating Platelet Aggregates by Exercise in Coronary Patients." *Circulation* 61 (1980): 62–65.
25. Sarajas, H. S. S. "Reaction Patterns of Blood Platelets in Exercise." *Advances in Cardiology* 18 (1976): 176–195.
26. Letcher, R. L.; Pickering, T. G.; Chien, S.; Laragh, J. H. "Effects of

Exercise on Plasma Viscosity in Athletes and Sedentary Normal Subjects." *Clinical Cardiology* 4 (1981): 172–179.

27. Williams, R. S.; Logue, E. E.; Lewis, J. L.; Barton, T.; Stead, N. W.; Wallace, A. G.; Pizzo, S. V. "Physical Conditioning Augments the Fibrinolytic Response to Venous Occlusion in Healthy Adults." *New England Journal of Medicine* 302 (1980): 987–991.

Chapter 6. The Magic Runner

1. Folkins, C. H.; Lynch, S.; Gardner, M. M. "Psychological Fitness as a Function of Physical Fitness." *Archives of Physical Medicine and Rehabilitation* 53 (1972): 503–508.
2. MacMannis, D. R. "Factors Influencing the Psychological Impact of Running." Ph.D. diss., California School of Professional Psychology, 1979.
3. Brown, R. S.; Ramirez, D. E.; Taub, J. M. "The Prescription of Exercise for Depression." *Physician and Sportsmedicine* 6, no. 12 (Dec. 1978): 34–45.
4. Andrew, G. M.; Oldridge, N. B.; Parker, J. O.; Cunningham, D. A.; Rechnitzer, P. A.; Jones, N. L.; Buck, C.; Kavanagh, T.; Shephard, R. J.; Sutton, J. R. "Reasons for Dropout from Exercise Programs in Postcoronary Patients." *Medicine and Science in Sports and Exercise* 13 (1981): 164–168.
5. Morgan, W. P.; Horstman, D. H.; Cymerman, A.; Stokes, J. "Exercise as a Relaxation Technique." *Primary Cardiology* 6 (Aug. 1980): 48–57.
6. Epstein, D. "The Psychological Effects of an Aerobic Fitness Program on Normal Adults." Ph.D. diss., Institute of Advanced Psychological Studies of Adelphi University, 1982.
7. Pitts, F. N. "Biochemical Factors in Anxiety Neurosis." *Behavioral Science* 16 (1971): 82–91.
8. Stern, M. J.; Cleary, P. "National Exercise and Heart Disease Project. Long-term Psychosocial Outcome." *Archives of Internal Medicine* 142 (1982): 1093–1097.
9. Heinzelmann, F.; Bagley, R. W. "Response to Physical Activity Programs and Their Effects on Health Behavior." *Public Health Reports* 85 (1970): 905–911.
10. Moore, M. "Endorphins and Exercise: A Puzzling Relationship." *Physician and Sportsmedicine* 10, no. 2 (Feb. 1982): 111–114.
11. See note 10.
12. Kosterlitz, H. W.; McKnight, A. T. "Endorphins and Enkephalins." *Advances in Internal Medicine* 26 (1980): 1–36.
13. Markoff, R. A.; Ryan, P. R.; Young, T. "Endorphins and Mood Changes in Long-distance Running." *Medicine and Science in Sports and Exercise* 14 (1982): 11–15.
14. Cover story. "Running: 'Unity with Nature.' " *MD* 23 (April 1979): 96–107.
15. Sheehan, G. A. *Doctor George Sheehan's Medical Advice for Runners.* Mountain View, Calif.: World Publications, 1978.
16. Deaton, J. "Run, Doctor, Run." *Physician's Management* 20 (Sept. 1980): 105–112.

17. Kostrubala, T., in Klinck, L. "Running: The New 'High.'" *Harper's Bazaar* (Sept. 1979): 151.
18. Switzer, K., in Christmyer, M. "Boston Marathon Has a Long History." *Forum on Medicine* (April 1978): 14–19.
19. Sheehan, G. A. "The Moral Equivalent of War." *Physician and Sportsmedicine* 8, no. 12 (Dec. 1980): 37.
20. Olsen, E. "The Fastest Woman on the Track." *The Runner* 3 (Aug. 1981): 24–30.
21. Ashford, E., in Olsen, E. See note 20.

Chapter 7. The Dangers of Exercise
1. Koplan, J. P.; Powell, K. E.; Sikes, R. K.; Shirley, R. W.; Campbell, C. C. "An Epidemiologic Study of the Benefits and Risks of Running." *Journal of the American Medical Association* 248 (1982): 3118–3121.
2. Clement, D. B.; Taunton, J. E.; Smart, G. W.; McNicol, K. L. "A Survey of Overuse Running Injuries." *Physician and Sportsmedicine* 9, no. 5 (May 1981): 547–558.
3. Berson, B. L.; Rolnick, A. M.; Ramos, C. G.; Thornton, J. "An Epidemiologic Study of Squash Injuries." *American Journal of Sports Medicine* 9 (1981): 103–106.
4. Nicholas, J. A. "Sports Medicine—Past, Present, and Future." *American Journal of Sports Medicine* 8 (1980): 389–394.
5. Cooper, K. H., in Long, C., ed. *Prevention and Rehabilitation in Ischemic Heart Disease.* Baltimore: Williams & Wilkins, 1980.
6. Brody, D.; Konecke, S.; Day, S. W.; Kryder, S. "A Study of 4,000 Running Injuries." *Running Times*, no. 54 (July 1981): 22–29.
7. Sheehan, G. A. "Downhill Demon." *Physician and Sportsmedicine* 9, no. 1 (Jan. 1981): 43.
8. See note 19, chapter 6.
9. Morgan, W. P. "Negative Addiction in Runners." *Physician and Sportsmedicine* 7, no. 2 (Feb. 1979): 57–70.
10. Kent, F. "Athletes Wait Too Long to Report Injuries." *Physician and Sportsmedicine* 10, no. 4 (April 1982): 127–129.
11. Fixx, James, at White House Symposium on Physical Fitness and Sports Medicine, Oct. 1980. *American Medical News* (31 Oct. 1980): 21.
12. See note 10.
13. See note 10.
14. *New York Times*, 20 April 1982. Confirmed in telephone conversation with author, 4 Oct. 1983.
15. Paris, S. *American Medical News* (23 May 1980): 13.
16. Haymond, T. *American Medical News* (23 May 1980): 13.
17. See note 16, chapter 6.
18. Sullivan, D. J. "Stress Fractures in Runners." Paper presented at meeting of the American College of Surgeons, Chicago, Oct. 1982.
19. Kiernan, H. A. *The Stethoscope* 35, no. 1 (Jan. 1980): 2. Published by Public Interest Dept. of The Presbyterian Hospital, New York, N.Y.
20. Sheffer, A. L.; Austen, K. F. "Exercise-induced Anaphylaxis." *Journal of Allergy and Clinical Immunology* 66 (1980): 106–111.

21. Elliot, Robert. Personal communication.
22. Waller, B. F.; Roberts, W. C. "Sudden Death While Running in Conditioned Runners Aged 40 Years or Over." *American Journal of Cardiology* 45 (1980): 1292–1300.
23. Noakes, T. D.; Opie, L. H.; Kleynhaus, P. H. T. "Autopsy-proved Coronary Atherosclerosis in Marathon Runners." *New England Journal of Medicine* 301 (1979): 86–89.
24. Virmani, R. "Jogging, Marathon Running, and Death." *Primary Cardiology* 8 (April 1982): 96–107.
25. Virmani, R.; Rabinowitz, M.; McAllister, H. A., Jr. "Nontraumatic Death in Joggers: A Series of 30 Patients at Autopsy." *American Journal of Medicine* 72 (1982): 874–882.
26. See note 24.
27. Thompson, P. D.; Stern, M. P.; Williams, M. S.; Duncan, K.; Haskell, W. L.; Wood, P. D. "Death During Jogging or Running." *Journal of the American Medical Association* 242 (1979): 1265–1267.
28. Handler, J. B.; Asay, R. W.; Warren, S. E.; Shea, P. M. "Symptomatic Coronary Artery Disease in a Marathon Runner." *Journal of the American Medical Association* 248 (1982): 717–719.
29. Opie, L. H. "Long Distance Running and Sudden Death." *New England Journal of Medicine* 293 (1975): 941–942.
30. Maron, B. J.; Roberts, W. C.; McAllister, H. A.; Rosing, D. R.; Epstein, S. E. "Sudden Death in Young Athletes." *Circulation* 62 (1980): 218–229.
31. See note 27.
32. Steward, D. G. "A New Perspective on Coronary Heart Disease." *Physician and Sportsmedicine* 8, no. 3 (March 1980): 171–174.
33. Noakes, T. D.; Opie, L. H. "Heart Disease in Marathon Runners." *Physician and Sportsmedicine* 7, no. 11 (Nov. 1979): 141–142.
34. French, A. J.; Dock, W. "Fatal Coronary Atherosclerosis in Young Soldiers." *Journal of the American Medical Association* 124 (1944): 1233–1237.
35. Moritz, A. R.; Zamcheck, N. "Sudden and Unexpected Deaths of Young Soldiers." *Archives of Pathology* 42 (1946): 459–494.
36. Yater, W. M.; Traum, A. H.; Brown, W. G.; Fitzgerald, R. P.; Geisler, M. A.; Wilcox, B. B. "Coronary Artery Disease in Men Eighteen to Thirty-nine Years of Age." *American Heart Journal* 36 (1948): 334–372, 481–526, 683–722.
37. Liberthson, R. R.; Nagel, E. L.; Hirschman, J. C.; Nussenfeld, S. R.; Blackbourne, B. D.; Davis, J. H. "Pathophysiologic Observations in Prehospital Ventricular Fibrillation and Sudden Cardiac Death." *Circulation* 49 (1974): 790–798.
38. Friedman, M.; Manwaring, J. H.; Rosenman, R. H.; Donlon, G.; Ortega, P.; Grube, S. M. "Instantaneous and Sudden Deaths." *Journal of the American Medical Association* 225 (1973): 1319–1328.
39. Thompson, P. D.; Funk, E. J.; Carleton, R. A.; Sturner, W. Q. "Incidence of Death During Jogging in Rhode Island from 1975 through 1980." *Journal of the American Medical Association* 247 (1982): 2535–2569.

40. Opie, L. H. "Sudden Death and Sport." *Lancet* 1 (1975): 263–266.
41. Shepard, A. J. "Sudden Death: A Significant Hazard of Exercise?" *British Journal of Sports Medicine* 8 (1974): 101–110.
42. Hossack, K. F.; Hartwig, R. "Cardiac Arrest During Cardiac Rehabilitation: Identification of High Risk Patients." *American Journal of Cardiology* 49 (1982): 915.
43. Gibbons, L. W.; Cooper, K. H.; Meyer, B. M.; Ellison, R. C. "The Acute Cardiac Risk of Strenuous Exercise." *Journal of the American Medical Association* 244 (1980): 1799–1801.
44. Vander, L.; Franklin, B.; Rubenfire, M. "Cardiovascular Complications of Recreational Physical Activity." *Physician and Sportsmedicine* 10, no. 6 (June 1982): 89–96.

Index

Addiction to exercise, 101–5
Aerobics, 19
  dancing, 130
Aerobics Research, Institute for, 119
Allergy to exercise, 107–8
American College of Cardiology, 37
American College of Sports Medicine, 74
American Heart Association, Committee on Exercise of the, 31, 40–41
American Journal of Cardiology, 66
Anaphylaxis, 107–8
Anemia, runner's (sports anemia), 108
Angina pectoris, 15, 16, 19, 24
Anxiety, exercise as therapy for, 84–85, 88–90
Archives of Internal Medicine, 90
Arrhythmias, 16, 36–37, 63, 116, 118
Arteries, coronary, 14–15
  atherosclerosis of. *See* Atherosclerosis.
  collateral blood vessels, 65–67
  disease risk factors, reduction of, 67–81. *See also* Coronary heart disease; *specific subjects*.
  hemostasis and, 76–81
  injuries to, 62, 78–79
  stress tests and, 31–32
Ashford, Evelyn, 96

Asthma, exercise-induced, 108
Atherosclerosis, 14, 24, 61–63
  as cause of death of runners, 112, 113
  injury to arteries and development of, 62, 78–79
  lipoproteins and, 72–76
Athlete's heart, 21

Bagley, Richard W., 91
Basketball, 123
Bassler, Dr. Thomas J., 50–51, 76, 111, 115
Bicycle testing, 26, 27. *See also* Stress tests and testing.
Bicycling, 130–31
Blood
  hemostatic system and, 76–81
  runner's anemia (sports anemia), 108
Blood pressure, 20
  hypertension and coronary disease, 67, 68, 69, 70–72
  stress testing and, 26, 28, 30, 32
Boston Marathon, 2, 103
British Heart Journal, 57–58
Brody, Dr. David M., 99, 100

Cable Health Network, 5
Calisthenics, 130

145

Hand-grip test, isometric, 26
Handler, Dr. Jeffrey B., 113–14
Harvard alumni, longevity study of, 50, 56
Hawaii, University of, 94
Health Insurance Plan of Greater New York, 49, 54–55, 56
Heart
blood flow. *See* Arteries, coronary.
diseases of. *See* Cardiovascular disorders; Coronary heart disease; *specific subjects.*
electrocardiograms of, 28–30, 32–33
fitness and, 14, 16–23
myocarditis, 109–10
rate, 18–21, 27–28, 126
rhythm, 36–37, 126–27. *See also* Arrhythmias.
stress testing and, 27–43. *See also* Stress tests and testing.
Heart attacks, 15–16, 24. *See also* Coronary heart disease.
blood clotting and, 76–78
danger of in exercise, 110–20
probability, statistical, among exercising population, 119–20
rehabilitation following, 63–65, 119, 133–34
risk of, reduction of, 67–81
Heatstroke, 107
Heinzelmann, Dr. Fred, 91
Hemostasis, 76–81
Heredity, longevity and, 46, 53
Hormones
changes in among women exercisers, 105–6
psychological responses to exercise and, 92–96
Hypertension, 67, 68, 69, 70–72. *See also* Blood pressure.
Hyperthermia, 107

Hypertrophic cardiomyopathy, 114–15
Hypothermia, 103, 107

Injuries and other hazards, 97
anaphylaxis, 107–8
avoidance of, 122–29
ignoring of and addiction to exercise, 101–5
menstruation, changes in, 105–6
orthopedic, 97–105
osteoporosis, 105, 106
thermal abnormalities, 103, 106–7
viral ailments, 109–10
warning signals, 111, 115, 123–27
women, 104–6
International Congress on Lipoproteins and Atherosclerosis, 75
Isometric hand-grip test, 26

Jane Fonda's Workout Book (Fonda), 3
Jogging and joggers, 1–2, 6, 7, 74, 78, 86, 99, 123. *See also* Running and runners.
coronary heart disease as cause of death of joggers, 113
incidence of death during jogging, 118
injuries, 101, 104. *See also* Injuries and other hazards.
Journal of the American Medical Association, 42

Kent, Fraser, 102
Keys, Ancel, 75–76
Kiernan, Dr. Howard A., 105

Lancet, 9
Lebow, Fred, 2, 103
L'Eggs Mini-Marathon, 2
Limits to exertion
setting personal, 122–29

Pittsburgh, University of, School of
  Medicine of, 75
Popularity and exploitation of exercising, 1–12
Programs, exercise
  supervised and/or organized, 4,
  124–25, 128–29
  tape cassettes, 130
  television programs, 130
Psychological responses to exercise,
  82–96
  anxiety and, 84–85, 88–90
  attitudes toward exertion and, 87–
  88
  depression and, 84–87, 89, 90
  diversion, 92
  endorphins and, 93–96
  mastery, sense of, 91–92
  runner's high, 94–96
  social interaction and, 90–91
Publications, popular, 3, 50
Public Health Reports, 91
Pulse, taking own, 126–27

Railroad workers, longevity studies
  of, 49, 53–54, 56–57
Risk factors of coronary disease, reduction of, 61–81
  cholesterol, 67–68, 72–76
  collateral coronary circulation, 65–
  67
  hemostasis and, 76–81
  hypertension, 67, 68, 69, 70–72
  lipoproteins, 72–76
  primary factors, 67–76
  primary prevention, 61–63
  secondary factors, 67
  secondary prevention, 62–65
  smoking, cigarette, 67–68, 69, 76,
  78
  tertiary prevention, 63, 65
Roberts, Dr. William C., 112
Rosenman, Dr. Ray H., 68

Runner, The, 50
Runners Handbook, 4
running and runners, 1–2, 6, 50–51,
  74, 76. *See also* Jogging and
  joggers; Marathon running and
  runners.
  addiction to, 101–4
  coronary heart disease, prevalence
  among runners, 112, 113, 114,
  115
  injuries and hazards, 97–116. *See
  also* Injuries and other hazards;
  specific subjects.
  injury, avoiding, 122–23
  runner's high, 94–96
  women, 104–6
Ryan, Jim, 103

Salazar, Alberto, 103
Sarajas, Dr. H. S. S., 80
Selection of exercise activity, 129–35
Self, 3
Sheehan, Dr. George, 22, 95, 101
Shorter, Frank, 50
Skiing injuries, 98, 102
  avoidance of, 122
Smoking, cigarette, and risk of coronary disease, 67–68, 69, 76,
  78
Squash injuries, 98
Stamler, Dr. Jeremiah, 69
Steward, Derek G., 115
Stress, mortality and, 46
Stress tests and testing, 9–11, 24–43
  bicycle, stationary exercise, 26, 27
  blood pressure and, 26, 28, 30, 32
  costs of, 10
  eating and, 32–33
  electrocardiograms, use of, 28–30,
  32–33
  end points of, 27–28
  environmental factors affecting results of, 41

Stress tests and testing, (*cont.*)
  as exercise guideline, 40–42
  fallibility of, 29–43
  financial aspects of, 10–11
  follow-up of abnormal results, 39–40
  hand-grip, isometric, 26
  as information source, additional, 37–38
  multistage, 26–31
  purposes of, 9–10, 25, 31
  reproducibility problems, 36–37, 39
  risks involved in, 42–43
  sensitivity of, 33–36
  single-stage, 25–26, 29
  treadmill, 26–27
  of women, 36
Sullivan, Dr. Dennis J., 104
Swimming, 129–30
Switzer, Kathy, 95

Taunton, Dr. J. E., 98, 99–100
Taylor, H. L., 49, 53–54
Television
  exercise programs, 130
  and popularization of exercise, 5
Tennis, dangers of, 98, 100
  avoidance of, 123
Thermal abnormalities, exertion and, 103, 106–7

Thompson, Dr. Paul D., 113, 114, 115
Toronto Western Hospital, 102
Training effect, 19–22
Transit workers, studies of London, 8–9, 48–49, 52–53, 59
Treadmill testing, 26–27. *See also* Stress tests and testing.
Triglycerides, lipoproteins and, 72

United States Air Force study, 36

Viral ailments, dangers of "working off," 109–10
Virmani, Dr. Renu, 112–13

Walking, as ideal exercise, 131–34
Waller, Dr. Bruce F., 112
Weight
  and longevity, 52
  loss, menstrual abnormalities and, 106
  and risk of coronary heart disease, 69
Wilhelmsen, Dr. L., 68–69
Women
  clothing, 7
  injuries and other hazards, 104–6
  statistical probability of cardiac events among exercisers, 119–20
  stress tests of, 36
World Health Organization, 64